New Age Biological Warfare
And
Pandemic

New Age Biological Warfare
And
Pandemic

Virus ....the Braham Astra

Lt Gen Virin Dhir

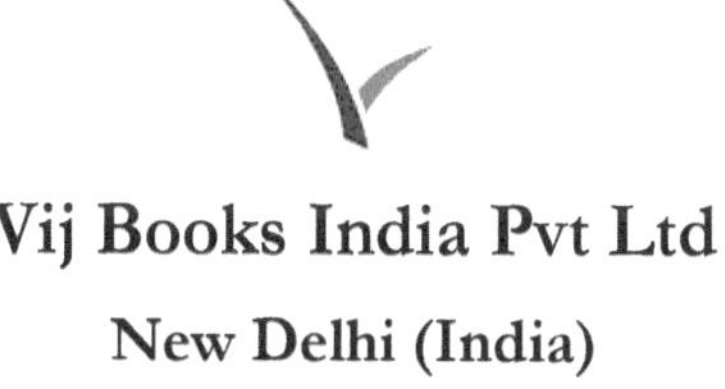

Vij Books India Pvt Ltd

New Delhi (India)

Published by

Vij Books India Pvt Ltd
(Publishers, Distributors & Importers)
2/19, Ansari Road
Delhi – 110 002
Phones: 91-11-43596460, 91-11-47340674
Mob: 9811094883
e-mail: contact@vijpublishing.com

Copyright © 2022, *Lt Gen Virin Dhir*

ISBN: 978-93-93499-16-5 (Hardback)
ISBN: 978-93-93499-17-2   (Paperback)
ISBN: 978-93-93499-22-6 (ebook)

All rights reserved.

No part of this book may be reproduced, stored in a retrieval system, transmitted or utilized in any form or by any means, electronic, mechanical, photocopying, recording or otherwise, without the prior permission of the copyright owner. Application for such permission should be addressed to the publisher.

The views expressed in the book are of author and not necessarily those of the Editors, or the publishers.

Dedicated to

Neeli - My Love

Viyan and Akshat – My world

From the Author

I am conscious of the fact that "New Age Biological Warfare and Pandemic – Virus …….. the Braham Astra" is perhaps the first book ever published in India covering different aspects of the biological warfare.

While carrying the burden of this honor, I humbly accept that there may be some gaps in presenting the subject. It always happens when you are the first one to pick up the hat!

Contents

From the Author		vii
Preface		xi
1.	History of Biological Warfare – *Disease as a Weapon of War*	1
2.	Biological Weapons – *The Silent Killers*	11
3.	Genetic Engineering – *The Game Changer*	25
4.	Strategic Thought – *Military Imperatives*	37
5.	Bioterrorism – *An Asymmetric Power Play*	54
6.	Bio Security – *The Challenges and Responses*	67
7.	Biological Warfare Programs of Major Powers - *An Open Secret*	78
8.	Biological and Toxin Weapons Convention 1972 - *Disarmament and Global Security*	93
9.	Covid-19 Pandemic – *The Virus Parade*	103
10.	Vaccine – *The Self Defense Armor*	116
11.	India and Pandemic – *Need for System Upgrade*	127
12.	What Lies Ahead…	141
Bibliography		147
Index		153

Preface

A narrative:

> "The world is in turmoil. Across a number of countries, millions of people are sick and there have been a large number of deaths. Medical facilities are overwhelmed: doctors and staff are in a state of exhaustion. National leadership is confused, and the devastation brooks no end".

In the past, you would have identified the above scenario as representing the aftermath of a major nuclear strike. But, cut to year 2020, and none would have any difficulty in pinning it down to the effects of the ongoing Covid-19 pandemic. The SARS CoV-2 virus has spared none and respected no boundaries between nations, rich and poor, people of colour and race – it has left the world "gasping for breath".

During the harrowing times of the pandemic, I undertook to design and develop a low-cost ventilator to assist delivery of Oxygen to the patients. This entailed a deep study of the coronavirus and genetic engineering. With my long years of service in the Indian Army, I could discern that the coronavirus had an overarching potential to be developed into a biological weapon. The extent of wrath suffered by the world was the clearest evidence that here was a biological weapon, which would completely transform biological warfare. That realization has been the trigger for me to write this book.

Since ancient times, biological weapons had been part of man's arsenal in the form of poisoned arrows, scorpion bombs and disease-causing germs. Even in modern times, these have been in prominence as part of the formidable triad of NBC (Nuclear, Biological and Chemical) warfare. There was a biological weapons backdrop to the Korean War, Vietnam War and the war in Iraq. In recent times, the bioterrorism events like that of Aum Shinrikyo in Japan and "Amerithrax" letters in the USA have confirmed the interest and competence of the non-state actors in this type of warfare. Biological warfare must become an integral part of strategic planning in national and international security domains with such threats looming on the horizon.

Three main factors underscore the recent overbearing impact of biological weapons on the strategic environment. First, the revolution in Biotechnology has created the means to modify the genome of a virus through genetic engineering. It is becoming possible to synthesize a pathogen, which is more transmissible and virulent.

Second, Covid-19 pandemic has demonstrated the destructive potential that the virus based biological weapons possess. The pandemic has caused disruptions and upheaval across the world – millions have died and many are suffering long term effects, an estimated loss of 3 to 4 trillion dollars has occurred to the global economy; industrial production and supply chains have been disturbed. Yet, the end to this misery is not in sight, with new mutations/variants of the virus continuing to appear in different places. The world has changed forever, having been exposed to "lockdowns" and "work from home".

Third, in terms of security, the future battle may no longer be fought on the frontiers alone. Biological weapons have the capacity to spread the battle spaces across the complete territory of a state. The boundaries between military and non-military resources, personnel and conduct of operations have been diffused. New strategic and operational concepts need to be evolved. It is not the "combat potential" of the defence forces alone but the "combined potential" of military and civil resources that will determine the path to victory. The latter will comprise the military and Paramilitary forces, civil disaster management agencies, Doctors and medical staff, public health agencies, scientists, the industry, the economy, policy planners, political leadership and even the NGOs.

The fact is that whatever is needed to fight a pandemic is equally good for military defence during a biological war. This has created an immense common space of integrated working between civil public health agencies and military resources. Hopefully, this book will arm all such "Bio Warriors" with adequate knowledge of important aspects of biological warfare and fighting a pandemic.

The book opens with the historical perspective of biological warfare starting from the ancient times. The next chapter covers the intrinsic aspects of biological weapons, including their classification into different categories and gives insight into the likelihood of SARS CoV-2 virus being a biological weapon. The following chapter highlights the ongoing revolution in Biotechnology. A game-changer, genetic engineering has now made it possible to modify or synthesize a pathogen genome; thus changing its characteristics manyfold. Literally speaking, the virus can now be structured to imbibe the power of a "Braham Astra".

The need for evolving new strategic concepts is highlighted in the next chapter. Propositions like: small weapon big bang, retaliatory assured destruction, fog of ambiguities and uncertainties, bio umbrella, multi-space battles have been discussed. This is followed by the study of Bio-Terrorism and asymmetric conflict, the space in which biological warfare is most likely to manifest.

The next chapter covers the many strands of biosecurity: biodefence preparedness, intelligence, trust and transparency, global cooperation and compliance, the safety of research laboratories, genetic research and threat assessment. These have to be strung together through strategy and systems to safeguard and protect a nation and its citizens against the catastrophic effects of a biological event.

The following chapter looks at the biological warfare programs being purportedly run by some states in violation of the international treaty. But, the treaty itself lacks strict verification and implementation mechanisms. This lackadaisical global effort at controlling the spread of biological weapons is discussed next under the Biological and Toxin Weapons Convention 1972.

Salient aspects of Covid-19 pandemic have been analyzed so as to evolve strategies to meet the challenges of a future pandemic to national security. Vaccines provide an effective defence against infectious diseases. Their development and trial process have been briefly explained. This would aid in appreciating the role of genetic engineering in future development of vaccines.

Finally, the context of biological events is brought closer home. India's systems and infrastructure to manage such disasters and emergencies are evaluated. Some recommendations for strengthening the same have been made.

The book ends with crystal gazing at what lies ahead. For sure, biological weapons remain a plausible threat in future, and the international community has to shoulder the task of safeguarding global security. One is reminded of the prophetic words of Bill Gates uttered in 2015:

> "If anything kills over 10 million people in the next few decades, it is likely to be a highly infectious virus, rather than a war."

History of Biological Warfare – *Disease as a Weapon of War*

Technology, disease and war have been part of the human story from time immemorial. In the early ages, the man used technology to make basic tools to ease his daily chores as well as he used arrows and spears for hunting food and for fighting his opponents. This dual use of technology found its parallel in disease too. The disease refers to any condition that causes dysfunction, pain, distress, disability, or death in humans and living organisms. It came naturally to the warriors to use disease as a weapon of war by spreading it amongst the enemy. And that marks the origin of Biological Warfare wherein the man found ways to use the spread of disease as a means to get the better of the enemy.

Before proceeding further, it may be proper to understand as to what constitutes Biological Warfare. In the past it has been a common practice to club together three forms of warfare, namely Nuclear, Biological and Chemical Warfare, commonly referred to by the acronym NBC. Although, all three involve use of weapons of mass destruction, it is time that these are treated as different entities as they differ vastly in concept, scope, conduct and destructive power.

Biological Warfare (BW for short) is the use of biological toxins or infectious agents such as bacteria, viruses, insects and fungi with the intent to kill, harm or incapacitate humans, animals or plants as an act of war. On the other hand, Chemical Warfare involves the use of chemicals to cause harm to the enemy. As regards Nuclear Warfare, it involves the use of nuclear weapons as part of the military and political strategies. Also, unlike Nuclear Warfare, Biological Warfare does not destroy physical structures and impacts only living beings.

For ease of understanding and also to maintain a relationship with impactful events, the historical perspective has been covered in distinct phases, beginning with the early ages.

Early Ages

Throughout history, humans have devised new ways to kill their opponents. When technology was primitive, they used easiest of the means like burning the crops to undermine an enemy. The infectious diseases were recognised for their weapon potential very early. The use of filth, cadavers and animal carcasses had devastating effects and weakened the enemy. Polluting of wells and other sources of water was a common strategy of war.

It is claimed that during the period 1500 – 1200 BCE, the victims of tularemia (rabbit fever) were driven into enemy lands to spread the disease. During the First Sacred War in Greece in about 590 BCE, Athens and Amphictionic League poisoned the water supply of the besieged city of Kirrha with the toxic plant hellebore. During 4th century BC, Scythian archers dipped their arrow tips into decomposing cadavers of humans or in blood mixed with dung: thus making these contaminated with dangerous bacterial agents. The Scythians were known for adding power to their usual weapons by using these as carriers of disease-causing agents as well as deadly poisons.

This strategy of polluting wells and other sources of water with infectious substances continued to be used in many European wars, the American Civil War and other conflicts.

Middle Ages

During the middle ages, the military leaders exploited the potential of using diseased cadavers and animal carcasses as biological weapons. In 1346, in the siege of Caffa, the Tartar forces hurled the bodies of victims of plague over the walls into the besieged city, thereby initiating plague outbreak. This incident is considered to be responsible for subsequent bubonic plague pandemic, known as Black Death, that swept through Europe, the Near East and North Africa during the 14 th century. It is the most fatal pandemic recorded in human history, causing the death of 75–200 million people.

Another incidence of throwing bodies of dead soldiers into enemy camps for causing disease happened in Karolstein Castle in 1422, including the attackers throwing 2000 carriage-loads of dung over the walls. The author has visited the Karolstein Castle during a tour of Europe. Militarily, it is a formidable structure, architecturally fascinating and technically, a brilliant piece of engineering. It would have been an insurmountable task for an attacker to gain access into the castle in the usual course.

Again in 1710, a similar strategy of catapulting cadavers of plague victims over the city walls of Reval was used during the battle between Swedish and Russian forces.

Another deadly disease "Smallpox" came to be used as a biological weapon. In 1754, Sir Jeffrey Amherst, the Commander of the British forces in North America suggested the deliberate and planned use of smallpox to demolish the native Indian population during the French – Indian wars. Accordingly, the natives were given blankets laden with smallpox, which resulted in an outbreak of smallpox among the Indian tribes in the Ohio River Valley.

Modern Age

With the development of modern microbiology as explained in the next Chapter, the isolation and production of stocks of specific pathogens became possible. Thus, 20th century saw the biological warfare becoming more sophisticated. During World War I, the Germans attempted to ship horses and cattle inoculated with disease producing bacteria, such as Bascillus Anthracis (anthrax) and Pseudomonas pseudomallei (glanders) to the United States and other countries. It is a different matter that this attempt did not produce any military success. In 1915, there was a German attempt to spread plague in St Petersburg in order to weaken Russian resistance. It appeared to be an act of desperation on part of German forces as their offensive was tottering.

World War I was followed in continuum by the influenza epidemic from 1918 – 20, also known as the Spanish Flu. It was caused by HINI virus and was the most severe pandemic accounting for nearly 50 million deaths. The high mortality in healthy people, including those in 20-40 years age group was a unique feature of this epidemic. With no vaccine to protect against influenza infection and no antibiotics to treat secondary infection, disease control efforts were limited to non-pharmaceutical interventions such as isolation, quarantine and good personal hygiene. While the Spanish Flu of 1917- 1918 has always been considered a natural calamity, the enormous loss of life left an indelible imprint on the minds of the strategists as to the harmful potential of a virus, a tiny pathogen. So, here was a future weapon of mass destruction that may become a reality with the advances in microbiology.

With the horrors of World War I fresh in their minds, most of the countries signed 1925 Geneva Protocol, which prohibited the use of Asphyxiating, Poisonous or other gases, and of Bacteriological methods of warfare. Unfortunately, this protocol said nothing about experimentation, production, storage or transfer aspects. Consequently, there was no check on the proliferation of activities related to biological weapons. However, 1925 protocol became a precursor to subsequent Biological and Toxin Weapons Convention 1972.

World War II

Despite signing the Geneva 1925 Protocol, several countries, including the United States, Belgium, Canada, Great Britain, Italy, the Netherlands, Poland, Japan, and the former Soviet Union, began to develop biological weapons.

Between 1932 and 1945, Japan's biological warfare program (called Unit 731) experimented with inoculation of agents causing anthrax, plague, cholera, gangrene and other highly infectious diseases. More than 10,000 prisoners are believed to have died as a result of this experimental inoculation of biological agents. Three veterans of Unit 731 testified in an interview in 1989 that they contaminated the Horustein river with typhoid pathogen near the Soviet troops during the Battle of Khalkhin Gol. In 1940, the Imperial Japanese Air Force bombed Ningbo with ceramic bombs full of fleas carrying the bubonic plague. Many of these operations were ineffective due to inefficient delivery systems, using disease-bearing insects rather than dispersing the agent as a bioaerosol cloud.

During the final stages of World War II, Japan had planned to use plague-based biological weapon against U.S.A. civilians in San Diego, California. The launch was set for September 22 1945 to dissuade America from attacking Japan. Eventually, this operation did not go through due to Japan's surrender on August 15 1945. In a verified testimony, link of Japan's biological weapons program was established with Noborito Institute.

While the Germans did not use biological agents against people, they did use these against the animals, infecting Allied horses with glanders and anthrax. The French also employed glanders against German horses.

Postwar Period

It has been said that, after the War, the USA enlisted some of the scientists from Noborito Institute of Japan to run a biological weapons project for the Korean War. In Britain, the 1950s saw the weaponisation of plague, brucellosis and tularemia viruses.

In 1948, during the Palestine War, International Red Cross reports raised suspicion that the Israeli Haganah militia had released Salmonella typhi bacteria into the water supply for the city of Acre. This caused an outbreak of Typhoid among the inhabitants. There were claims of attempt to poison the wells in Gaza.

During the Korean War, China and North Korea claimed that the USA had used biological weapons against them. It was alleged that M114 bursting bomb lets, containing agent brucellosis, in M33 cluster bombs were dropped. The North Korean Government made the allegations at the United Nations that biological weapon attacks had been made against them. Though the US denied the charges, they had the capability to undertake such attacks. As regards the method of dissemination, it was claimed based on certain evidence that mostly spraying was used. Another munition mentioned was air-bursting variable-time fuse leaflet bombs for insect dissemination.

Vietnam War

In comparison to chemical weapons in Vietnam, the use of biological weapons was less in volume and effect. There have been specific allegations that biological weapons were used against vegetation in Cham Thanh district of Tan province where all the rice, plants, fruit trees and orchards in a band of 2 kilometers were destroyed.

After the Vietnam War ended, there was an overwhelming sentiment and public outcry against the use of biological agents in war. In a major development, in 1969, President Richard Nixon through an executive order stopped production of biological weapons in the USA and allowed only scientific research of lethal biological agents and defensive measures such as immunisation and biosafety. The order mandated the cessation of offensive biological weapons research and production; and the destruction of the biological weapons arsenal. Signing of the Biological and Toxin Weapons Convention in 1972 followed this.

Laos Cambodia

In the late 1970s, there were allegations that planes and helicopters delivering aerosols of different colors attacked the inhabitants of Laos and Kampuchea. Many people who were exposed became disoriented and ill. These attacks were commonly described as "yellow rain." In fact it was highly controversial whether these clouds truly represented biological warfare agents. Some of these clouds were believed to comprise trichothecene toxins.

It is alleged that erstwhile Soviet Union supplied biological weapons, mainly fungal toxins (Mycotoxins) to government forces, to kill dissident tribal people and enemy soldiers in Laos, Cambodia and Afghanistan. Though the Soviet Government denied the charges, former US Secretary Alexander Haig on September 13 1981 claimed that sufficient evidence was available in support of this assertion.

Iraq - Weapons of Mass Destruction

In his quest for weapons of mass destruction, Saddam Hussein initiated an extensive biological weapons program in Iraq in the early 1980s. Details of this program surfaced only in the wake of Gulf war

(1990-91) following investigation conducted by the United Nations Special Commission (UNSCOM). Despite being a signatory to BWC 1972, the representatives of the Iraqi government announced to the Commission Team that they had conducted research into the offensive use of *B. anthracis* and botulinum toxins. This open admission of biological warfare research verified many of the concerns of the US intelligence community.

Iraq had extensive research facilities at Salman Pak and other sites, many of which were destroyed during the war. In 1995, further information on Iraq's offensive program was made available to United Nations inspectors. Field trials were conducted and biological agents were tested in various delivery systems, including rockets, aerial bombs, and spray tanks. In December 1990, the Iraqis filled 100 R400 bombs with botulinum toxin, 50 with anthrax, and 16 with aflatoxin. In addition, 13 Al Hussein (Scud) warheads were filled with botulinum toxin. Since, no actual biological attack took place, the conjecture is that the threat of massive retaliation by the USA dissuaded Iraq.

Covert Assassinations

During 1970s, biological weapons were used for covert assassinations. In 1978, a Bulgarian exile named Georgi Markov was attacked and killed in London. This assassination later became known as the "umbrella killing", because weapon used was a device disguised as an umbrella. This weapon discharged a tiny pellet containing the toxin ricin. The pellet got embedded in Markov's leg tissues and he died within three days of the attack. A similar attempt to kill another Bulgarian exile occurred in Paris. In later years, it was revealed that the assassinations were carried out by the Communist Bulgarian Secret service with the technology procured from the Soviet Union.

Sverdlovsk Incident

During April 1979, an epidemic of anthrax occurred among the citizens of Sverdlovsk, Soviet Union. The epidemic occurred among people who lived and worked near a Soviet military microbiology facility. Many livestock died of anthrax in the same area, up to a distance of 50 km. The Soviet Union maintained that the anthrax outbreak was caused by the consumption of contaminated meat that was purchased on the black market. However, later in May 1992, Yeltsin admitted that the facility had been part of an offensive biological weapons program and that the epidemic was caused by an accidental release of anthrax spores.

Later, a report in 1995 stated that the Russian biological warfare program continued to exist after the 1979 incident. It employed about 25,000 to 30,000 people as part of Biopreparat project.

Religious Sects and Cults

Some religious sects have resorted to the violent use of biological agents to inflict panic among the public and to promote their cause and sphere of influence. One incident relates to the intentional contamination of salad bars in restaurants in Oregon by Rajneesh cult during September 1984. A total of 751 cases of severe enteritis were reported, and Salmonella typhimurium was identified as the causative organism. The follow up investigation could not conclusively identify the origin of the epidemic. However, in 1985, a member of the cult confirmed that it was a deliberate biological attack.

On March 18, 1995 the members of the Aum Shinrikyo cult in Japan attacked the Tokyo subway system with sarin gas. It resulted in killing 12 train passengers and injuring more than 5,000 people. The investigation into the incident disclosed evidence of a rudimentary biological weapons program. It was claimed that even before March 1995, the cult had attempted three unsuccessful biological attacks in Japan using anthrax and botulinum toxin.

Amerithrax

Seven days after the terrorist attacks of September 11, 2001 on the World Trade Centre, few anonymous letters laced with deadly anthrax spores began arriving at media companies and congressional offices in the USA. Over the ensuing months, five people died from inhaling anthrax and 17 others were sickened after exposure. It led to great fear and confusion among the public, and overwhelming workload on the public health agencies. The FBI conducted a seven yearlong investigation into the worst biological attack in the US history and it was codenamed " Amerithrax". It concluded that the attacker was Dr. Bruce Ivins of the US Army Medical Research Institute of Infectious

Diseases. Dr. Ivnis committed suicide before he could be charged. Anyway, this incident played a profound role in raising concerns over possible terrorist attacks using biological agents.

Covid -19 Pandemic

The COVID-19 pandemic is an ongoing pandemic caused by severe acute respiratory syndrome coronavirus 2 (SARS-Cov-2). The novel virus was identified in Wuhan, China, in December 2019. A number of variants of the disease have emerged and it has since spread globally, mostly through aerosol transmission. So far, more than 220 million cases and 5.60 million deaths have been confirmed, making it one of the deadliest pandemics in the history. Further, it has resulted in severe global social and economic disruption, leading to wide spread supply shortages. A massive vaccination program has been started worldwide to combat the spread of disease. The origin of the Corona virus has not been conclusively established so far.

Biotechnology Revolution

Since 1970s, there have been remarkable advances in techniques and applications of biotechnology, so much so that many expect 21st Century to be the "Biotechnology Century". The genome mapping and gene splicing is becoming commonplace. It will permit the development of a new class of biological agents engineered to elicit novel effects; thus providing new use options and expanding the biological warfare paradigm. While, these will not replace the traditional biological agents such as anthrax, but it will greatly enlarge the arsenal.

Latest advances in life sciences and molecular genetics, while serving humanity in finding cure to diseases like cancer, have the potential to raise the destruction quotient of the biological warfare many notches up.

Take Aways

Above review beginning with pre-historic times and leading up to current global turmoil caused by the pandemic, underscores the importance that the states need to accord to biosecurity. While the use of biological weapons may not have resulted in great victories, but these had an overwhelming psychological impact on the adversary. Some take aways from the review are mentioned below:

- It is a fact of history that virtually no nation capable of developing weapons of mass destruction has ever abstained from doing so. It applies equally well in the case of biological warfare.

- It is difficult to differentiate between a naturally occurring epidemic and a biological warfare attack. This enables deniability and secrecy.

- Due to time delay in spread of disease, it becomes difficult to trace the origin of a biological agent. This attribute makes it a handy weapon for non-state actors enabling them to make good their escape.

- Though many state and non-state actors acquire access to the relevant technology, the process of weaponisation is an intricate one, a factor that has been instrumental in limiting the proliferation of biological weapons.

- Biological weapons are a great equaliser in an asymmetric hostile situation. Iraq embarked upon an extensive biological warfare program to produce its own weapons of mass destruction in order to pose a threat to the mighty USA.

- Biological weapons cover a wide spectrum of usage from use against an individual, as in covert assassinations, to use as a weapon of mass destruction.

- There have been flagrant violations of BWTC, 1972. Many signatory countries have violated the treaty in the absence of stringent punitive measures.

- Total transformation of biological warfare is on the way in the 21st Century on account of stupendous advances in biotechnology. Genetically engineered pathogens which are highly infectious and precise will make biological weapons much more potent.

Biological Weapons – *The Silent Killers*

Throughout history, natural diseases have played an overwhelming role in deciding the course of many battles. It is believed that Alexander the Great was killed by malaria at the height of his power. During the Walcheren Expedition, Napoleon flooded the Holland countryside to allow malaria to become rampant. He reportedly stated: "We must oppose the English with nothing but fever, which will soon devour them all." In World War II, Gen Douglas MacArthur's predicament in May 1943 was: "This will be a long war if for every division I have facing the enemy I must count on a second division in hospital with malaria and a third division convalescing from this debilitating disease".

Therefore, the military strategists have invariably thought about employing infectious diseases as a weapon of war. Disease-causing element is known by different names like: germ, pathogen, toxin, agent etc. Particular arrangements have to be made to deliver the pathogen into enemy territory and to ensure the spread of the disease. Thus:

> *"Biological weapons deliver toxins and microorganisms such as viruses and bacteria, so to deliberately inflict disease among people, animals and agriculture. Biological attacks can result in destruction of crops, temporarily discomforting a small community and killing large number of people."*

Biological Weapon – A Weapon of Mass Destruction (WMD)

Biological weapons like chemical weapons and nuclear weapons are commonly referred to as weapons of mass destruction. A biological warfare attack can potentially result in an epidemic or pandemic, there by creating a massive disruption in the society and posing serious challenges to the health authorities. But, biological weapons differ from other WMDs in many ways. First, the effects of a biological attack can take several days to appear which makes it difficult to anticipate and respond. Second, unlike other WMDs, biological weapons can only target the living beings i.e. humans, crops and animals and have no impact on infrastructure or equipment. Finally, unlike nuclear weapons, a biological weapons program does not usually require high-end technical inputs and significant financial investments. This puts the biological weapon capability within reach of smaller states and non-state actors.

The conventional weapons and nuclear weapons when employed, are accompanied by a burst and loud noise of the explosion. However, in the case of biological weapons employment, the whole operation can be carried out in silence and secrecy – hence the epithet *"the silent killers"*.

Constituents of a Biological Weapon System

Biological weapons are unique in their ability to inflict a large number of casualties over a wide area with minimal logistic requirements and by means, which can be virtually untraceable. The ease and low cost of producing an agent, the difficulty in detecting its presence and the potential to selectively target humans, animals, or plants make biological weapons a sought after choice.

A biological weapon has three components: a biological agent, some stability inducing additives promoting the dissemination and a delivery system. Each of these components presents a complex set of requirements and entails a number of complicated steps to arrive at the final configuration. For instance, in the case of a biological agent, the suitable agent has to be identified, its virulent strain obtained, and mass production undertaken, followed by its storage and packaging.

Biological Agents

Biological agents lie at the heart of biological weapons. It is essential to understand their characteristics, which form the basis for selecting a particular agent for a specific mission. Also, based on their harm potential, military suitability etc., the agents have been assigned different classifications. All such aspects are discussed in detail, as these have a bearing on developing strategic concepts and biosecurity.

Characteristics of Biological Agents

Although there are more than 1,200 biological agents that could be used to cause illness or death, relatively few possess the necessary characteristics to make them ideal candidates for biological warfare or terrorism agents. Various characteristics of agents that influence their suitability as biological weapons are stated below:

- ➢ **Virulence**. It reflects the relative severity of disease produced by the particular agent. Different microorganisms and different strains of the same organisms may cause diseases of different severity.

- ➢ **Infectivity**. It is indicative of the relative ease with which microorganisms establish themselves in a host species. Pathogens with high infectivity cause disease with relatively few organisms and vice a versa. One must know that high infectivity does not necessarily mean that the symptoms of disease appear more quickly, nor that the illness is more severe.

- ➢ **Pathogenicity**. It is the capability of an infectious agent to cause disease in a susceptible host.

- ➢ **Toxicity**. It is the relative severity of illness or incapacitation produced by a toxin.

- ➢ **Incubation Period**. It is the time between exposure to the infectious agent and the appearance of symptoms of the disease. The dose, virulence, route of entry and immunological factors of the host govern it.

- ➢ **Transmissibility**. Some biological agents may be transmitted from person-to-person directly, while others may involve indirect transmission through vectors. This factor has a bearing on casualty management.

- ➢ **Lethality**. It is the relative ease with which an agent can cause death in a susceptible population.

> **Stability**. It is the extent to which the viability of an agent is affected by various environmental factors like temperature, relative humidity, sunlight etc. A quantitative measure of stability is an agent's decay rate.

> **Other Factors**. These may include ease of production, stability when stored or transported and ease of dissemination.

Medical Classification of Biological Agents

Medical classification of biological agents is important to medical services in terms of detection, identification, prophylaxis, and treatment. Biological agents, which may be used as weapons, can be classified as follows:

> **Bacteria**. These are microscopic, single-celled organisms that exist in their millions, in every environment, both inside and outside other organisms. Some bacteria are harmful, but most serve a useful purpose. They reproduce by simple divisions. The diseases they produce often respond to specific therapy with antibiotics.

> **Viruses**. Virus is an extremely small entity, which is not fully acknowledged as living organism as it cannot survive outside a host. They require living cells in which to replicate. The diseases they produce do not generally respond to antibiotics.

> **Rickettsiae**. These are microorganisms, which have characteristics common to both bacteria and viruses. They are found in ticks, lice, fleas, mites and mammals. They are susceptible to broad-spectrum antibiotics.

> **Fungi**. These are primitive plants, which do not utilise photosynthesis and draw nutrition from decaying vegetable matter. They may be unicellular or filamentous and reproduce by means of spores. Fungi diseases may respond to various antimicrobial.

> **Toxins**. These are poisonous substances produced and derived from living plants, animals, or microorganisms. Some toxins may also be produced or altered by chemical actions.

Thus, the biological agents are of two main types: pathogens and toxins. Pathogens are disease-causing organisms and they have a self-replication property, which enables them to act at low concentrations and to keep spreading long after the attack. Pathogens include Bacteria (which can cause diseases such as plague or anthrax), Rickettsia, Viruses, and Fungi (which can cause crops' diseases like rice blast or cereal rust). Toxins, on the other hand, are poisonous substances produced by living things like snakes, insects, spiders, plants, etc. Although toxins are not self-replicating, their toxic power is high, and they are extremely lethal even in small quantities.

Public Health (CDC) Classification of Agents

A widely recognised public health classification of biological agents is the one defined by the U.S.A. Centre for Disease Control (CDC). It has concluded that the U.S.A. public health system and primary healthcare providers must be prepared to address varied biological agents, including pathogens that are rarely seen in the U.S.A.

CDC has stated that high priority agents include organisms that pose a risk to national security because they:

> ➢ Can be easily disseminated or transmitted person-to-person;

> ➢ Cause high mortality, with potential for major public health impact;

> ➢ Might cause public panic and social disruption; and

> ➢ Require special action for public health preparedness.

There are many different ways to categorise biological weapons according to lethality. The CDC divides them into three main categories: Category A, Category B, and Category C.

The Category A weapons are high-priority agents include organisms that pose a risk to national security because they can be easily disseminated or transmitted person-to-person; cause high mortality, with potential for major public health impact; might cause public panic and social disruption; and require special action for public health preparedness. They include:

- ➤ Variola major (smallpox);

- ➤ *Bacillus anthracis* (Anthrax);

- ➤ *Yersinia pestis* (plague);

- ➤ *Clostridium botulinum* toxin (botulism);

- ➤ *Francisella tularensis* (tularaemia);

- ➤ Filoviruses,

  - Ebola hemorrhagic fever,

  - Marburg hemorrhagic fever

- ➤ Arenaviruses.

Category B agents include biological weapons that are moderately easy to disseminate; cause moderate morbidity and low mortality; and require specific enhancements of CDC's diagnostic capacity and enhanced disease surveillance. They include:

- ➤ *Coxiella burnetti* (Q fever);

- ➤ *Brucella* species (brucellosis);

- ➤ *Burkholderia mallei* (glanders);

- ➤ Alpha viruses,

  - Venezuelan encephalomyelitis,

  - Eastern and western equine encephalomyelitis;

- ➤ Ricin toxin from *Ricinus communis* (castor beans);

- ➤ Epsilon toxin of *Clostridium perfringens*;

- ➤ *Staphylococcus* enterotoxin B.

Category C agents have third priority and include emerging pathogens that could be engineered for mass dissemination in the future because of their availability; ease of production and dissemination; and potential for high morbidity and mortality and major health impact. The preparedness for Category C agents requires ongoing research to improve disease detection, diagnosis, treatment, and prevention. They include:

- ➢ Nipah virus,

- ➢ Hantaviruses,

- ➢ Tick-borne hemorrhagic fever viruses,

- ➢ Tick-borne encephalitis viruses,

- ➢ Yellow fever and multidrug-resistant tuberculosis.

Military Classification

While the civil classification of biological agents is based on their connect with public health preparedness, in the case of military, the classification of agents is done based on their offensive employment. Therefore, the biological agents are classified in military terms of tactical, operational and strategic purposes.

Classification by Target

There is yet another classification of biological agents as per the target that they are employed against namely: anti –personal, anti-crop and anti- livestock.

Agents – Suitable for Building Biological Weapons

Mentioned below are some of the biological agents, which are considered suitable for building biological weapons. The factors considered are their characteristics, ease of production and amenability to safe handling.

- ➢ **Bacillus Anthracis (Anthrax).** A bacteria which causes Anthrax, it is one of the most deadly agent for use as a biological weapon. The gram-positive, rod shaped anthrax spores are found naturally in soil, can be produced in a laboratory, and last for a long time in the environment. It can be mixed with powders, sprays, food and water. The invisible, infectious, odorless and tasteless spores make Anthrax a flexible biological weapon.

- ➢ **Botulinum toxin**. This agent is relatively easy to produce and has extreme potency and lethality. Botulism is a serious muscle-paralysing disease caused by these bacteria, which can be found naturally in forest soils, and bottom sediments of lakes and streams. A Japanese biological warfare group is known to have infected war prisoners with C botulinum toxins during the occupation of Manchuria in World War II.

- ➢ **Variola major (Smallpox).** This virus causes Smallpox, a highly contagious and infectious disease that has no cure and can only be prevented by vaccination. It is believed that the Smallpox was used as a biological weapon against Native Americans.

  The Soviet government commenced a program in 1980 to develop smallpox virus in large quantities stored in refrigerated tanks to use as a biological weapon agent.

- ➢ **Francisella tularensis (Tularemia).** Extreme infectiousness, ease of dispersion, and ability to cause illness and death make Francisella tularensis bacterium a dangerous biological weapon. People affected with Francisella tularensis experience symptoms including skin ulcer, fever, cough, vomiting and diarrhoea. Dr Alibek, after defection to the West, has revealed that the Soviet Red Army used Tularensis against German troops in the battle of Stalingrad during World War II.

Biological Weapons – Delivery System

A biological agent alone cannot be termed a weapon; after adding some additives to stabilise it, a delivery system is required to get it to the target. Biological agents can be disseminated as aerosols, within food or water, by a zoonotic vector (rodent, insect), or by injection. The choice of a particular delivery system is guided by various military considerations.

Means of Delivery

Following means of delivery of biological agents are available:

> ➤ **Aerosol Sprays**. The airborne pathogen is dispersed as fine particles. To be infected, a person must breathe a sufficient quantity of particles into the lungs to cause the illness.

> ➤ **Explosion Delivery.** The use of an explosive device (bombs, grenades, special bullets) to deliver and spread biological agents is not as effective as the delivery by aerosol. This is because the bulk of the agent tends to be destroyed by the blast, leaving a small quantity capable of causing the disease.

> ➤ **Mixed with Food or Water**. Though an effective means of delivery, it will usually require large quantity of the agent so that end delivery to the target is in sufficient quantity.

> ➤ **Through the Skin**. In this case, the agent is absorbed or injected through the skin. It may be an ideal method for assassination but is not likely to be used to cause mass casualties.

Aerosol is the most common method of delivery used in biological weapons. Aerosol dispersal can be achieved using various spray devices. However, factors like wind speed, humidity, or sunlight may have to be taken into consideration. New technologies are facilitating effective cushioned delivery through artillery projectiles and missiles. Also, unmanned aerial vehicles (UAVs) in conjunction with precision-guided munitions offer an attractive means of delivery.

Miscellaneous Aspects

Biological Agents vs. Chemical Agents

There is often some confusion between biological and chemical agents. The Chemical Warfare involves the use of chemical agents. These agents like mustard gas or Agent Orange are used to incapacitate personnel by poisoning, burning, or asphyxiation.

The Biological Warfare involves the use of germ related weapons to cause disease. Biological agents include bacteria, viruses, fungi, and toxins. These have the ability to adversely affect human health in a variety of ways, ranging from relatively mild, allergic reactions to serious medical conditions—even death.

Bhopal gas tragedy was the result of accidental release of a poisonous gas at the Union Carbide plant. If used for military purpose, it woulds be called a chemical agent.

Biological agents can reproduce themselves inside the victim: usually they have a delayed effect and are hard to detect in the environment. It is hard to distinguish between a natural epidemic and a biological attack. On the other hand chemical agents are usually nauseating and can be detected in the environment.

Inherent Problems of Biological Weapons

A major problem with the biological weapons concerns the phenomenon of blow back i.e. the pathogen infecting the attacker's own troops. Since, there is no control over the flow of the pathogen, in aerosol form, in terms of its direction and the space it covers, there is likelihood that it may infect and harm own troops and civil population.

There are examples in history highlighting the blow back of the biological agent. During World War II, the Japanese had attacked the Chinese targets with plague-infected fleas being dropped from the aircrafts. While thousands of Chinese died during these biological attacks, it is reported that nearly 1000 Japanese troops operating in the area died due to the same. So, the biological weapons can act like double-edged sword.

Presently, there is no solution to the blow back issue; but through genetic engineering some options are being generated whereby the effects of the bio strike can be made selective or specific.

Scientific Advancements

Recent advances in biotechnology and the breakthroughs in gene editing are opening new windows in health management, but at the same time these are raising fresh concerns about weaponising of pathogens. Using gene-editing tools, including CRISPR, scientists are now able to modify an organism's DNA more efficiently, flexibly, and accurately than ever before.

As discussed in the preceding chapter, the Gene-editing techniques such as CRISPR could make biological weapons more deadly. It would be possible to develop novel or modified pathogens that would spread in a faster manner, infect more people, cause severe sickness, or resist treatment. The equipment needed for wide-area dispersal may become less necessary, for example, if a pathogen can be engineered to spread faster on its own. Even ways of tackling blow back problem are being worked upon.

"New Age Technologies" are ushering in a new era in development of biological weapons. In the past, the traditional genetic engineering techniques were tedious and laborious. All this has now changed. Not only can the required attributes of the agent be amplified, but also the scale in production can be achieved. The high pace of advances, in molecular sciences and genetics, is pushing the biological weapons to the centre stage.

Considerations – Resources and Cost

In the ambit of WMDs, compared to the cost of a nuclear weapon, biological weapons are extremely cheap. It is for this reason that the biological weapons are often referred to as poor man's atom bomb. An old analysis gives comparative cost ratio as 800 : 1 between nuclear weapons and the biological weapon. It is worth noting that Covid-19 responsible for millions of deaths has been caused by a miniscule quantity of SARS CoV-2 virus.

Nuclear weapons program require great deal of material resources and scientific effort. Even after manufacture, these have to be stored in safe bombproof silos. On the other hand, biological weapons can be produced in a dual-use facility with a reasonable affordability tag. Depending on method of deployment, these agents can be stored in an innocuous manner in ordinarily safe places.

Virus – the Braham Astra

The threat of use of biological agents on both military forces and the civil population is more likely now than at any other point in history. Though theoretically, any of the agents based on bacteria, virus, fungi, toxins could be used to develop a biological weapon, but the recent advances in life sciences have pushed the case up in favour of using virus-based agents.

CRISPR technology has become the technique of choice for gene editing, the latter being the tool to develop future biological weapons. However, the use of CRISPR on bacteria has been limited. Many bacteria do not possess robust DNA repair system, which reduces the efficacy of gene-editing techniques. On the other hand, the viruses can be genetically engineered or modified with due process stability.

The self-multiplication capability is much more pronounced in he virus as compared to the bacteria. This property is important to ensure fast spread of the disease.

Synthetic biology is making possible the development of novel viruses abinitio. Recently, the research team at the State University of New York had synthesised the poliovirus from scratch. In future, the molecular sciences hold the prospect of developing virus-based pathogens imbibing the desired military attributes.

A serious study of the scientific literature suggests that the virus-based weapons would act as the main stay of biological warfare and demonstrative effect of Covid-19 pandemic further adds to this observation. Going ahead "Virus……… The Braham Asrtra" may prove to be the proper aphorism.

SARS CoV-2 – A Biological Weapon?

Following the onslaught of Pandemic-19, many have raised the question whether SARS CoV-2 virus is a biological weapon. Many experts have examined the issue and the general view is that as of now SARS CoV-2 was not developed as a biological weapon. But, most of the observations made by the experts are nuanced and therefore the doubts still persist.

As known, SARS CoV-2 probably emerged and infected humans through an initial small-scale exposure in Wuhan, China around November 2019. Till date, the exact origin of the coronavirus has not been conclusively established. China has stonewalled detailed scientific investigation. One point generally agreed by the scientists is that SARS CoV-2 is not genetically engineered.

A novel coronavirus, SARS CoV-2 is a new strain of coronavirus that has not been previously identified in humans. It may have occurred through natural zoonotic transfer from bats to animals to humans. Further, different mutations of the coronavirus viz: Alpha, Beta, Gamma and Delta are quite consistent with the natural evolution. Therefore, Covid-19 pandemic caused by SARS CoV-2 virus may be a natural occurrence.

On the other hand, SARS CoV-2 virus has many attributes, which make it a good candidate to be developed into a formidable biological weapon. These include high infectiousness, virulence and transmissibility. Could it be that the Chinese researchers were undertaking scientific work on SARS CoV-2 virus, when its accident release happened? This theory has some circumstantial support; the initial start of the pandemic has taken place in close proximity of Wuhan Institute of Virology, China. This institute is reported to be working on military projects in conjunction with People's Liberation Army Medical Institute Therefore, the possible connection of the pandemic with the virus being a potential biological weapon cannot be ruled out.

If nothing else, the misery unleashed by SARS CoV-2 virus is a harsh reminder of the vulnerabilities of the society to the use of biological weapons. Also, the potential users of the biological weapons, which include rogue states and terrorist groups, have observed this display of the might of the virus. The new age biological weapons are likely to add another dimension to the national security domain.

To Conclude

Humans are not the only potential targets for future biological weapons. Both crops and livestock have been subjects of biological weapons research. Biological weapons against crops and animals could prove a very effective way of conducting war by causing famines and destabilising economies. Moreover, it may be easier to disguise their use as a natural event and could be combined with the attacks on human beings.

The biological weapons also represent an area where the rapid pace of technological change is having a major impact. Their capabilities in terms of destructive power and means of deployment are getting transformed. In the coming decades, new range of biological weapons may become available.

In view of the devastation caused by the Pandemic 19, the world is expected to become more sensitive to possession of biological weapons. It is expected that stricter curbs and stiff international controls may be implemented through BTWC 1972.

Genetic Engineering – *The Game Changer*

The revolution in Biotechnology is being considered as one of the most striking happening of the 21st Century. Rapid advances are taking place in molecular genetics and allied life sciences. Scientists are working on many fronts like finding cures for diseases like Cancer, stem cell therapies, organ transplants and developing a treatment for various genetic diseases. The technologies which were earlier the preserve of highly sophisticated laboratories, because of knowledge, costs and high-end equipment, are being replaced by alternate technologies which are easier to handle and require lesser resources.

One such discipline where the profound impact of advances in life sciences is being felt pertains to Biological Warfare. Till the nineteenth century, biological weapons development depended on natural pathogens. However, the scene altered dramatically from mid-twentieth century onwards. The revolution in Biotechnology has given the conventional biological warfare agents a new meaning - opening up the possibilities of genetically engineered pathogens being deployed as biological weapons.

It is not hard to imagine how some of these technologies could be used to develop more potent biological weapons. Some of these projects are able to overcome the current scientific and technological limits in the military use of pathogenic agents. A transformation in biological warfare is underway consequent to the advancements in life sciences and molecular genetics.

Biological systems are marked by their modular structure, which opens up the possibility of tinkering with individual elements. Such structural changes in sub-systems eventually reflect in big underlying changes that are made to happen in the overall system performance. Gene is the smallest unit like an atom in physics and provides this modularity. The genetic material (DNA or RNA) of a system, which contains all the information to control its functioning, can be removed from one pathogen and inserted into another as a means of altering its function. Modularity provides a degree of predictability in altered systems, and also enables altering their functions and performance.

Biotechnology and genetic engineering are relatively new fields of science. Since, many readers may not be familiar with the nature and scope of Biotechnology and genetic engineering, some details of these subjects are covered in the succeeding text.

Biotechnology

Biotechnology is the field that exploits living organisms to make technological advances in various fields for the sustainable development of mankind. It may be noted that such processes of living organisms have been used for more than 6,000 years to make essential products like bread, cheese, alcohol etc. It is just that the scientific field of microbiology did not exist at that time and hence the scientific understanding of the molecular processes was lacking. Modern biotechnology started in 1970s when it was primarily used for food processing and agriculture industries.

The concept of biotechnology encompasses a wide range of procedures for modifying living organisms according to human purposes, going back to domestication of animals, cultivation of the plants, and "improvements" to these through breeding programs that employ artificial selection and hybridisation. Modern usage also includes genetic engineering as well as cell and tissue culture technologies. Biotechnology has applications in four major areas, including health care (medical), crop production and agriculture, non-food (industrial) uses of crops and other products (e.g. biodegradable plastics, vegetable oil, biofuels), and environmental uses.

Colour Classification of Biotechnology

Depending upon the nature of the application, the field of biotechnology has been broken down into sub-disciplines. These are referred to as:

> Red Biotechnology – Used in medical process to produce new drugs and vaccines.

Green Biotechnology – Involves agricultural processes to produce pest-resistant crops and producing disease-resistant animals.

Blue Biotechnology – involves processes related to marine life.

Yellow Biotechnology – Involves processes related to food production like fermentation of cheese or alcohol.

Blue Biotechnology – It relates to the marine based resources.

Gold Biotechnology – It refers to the use of data, analytics and computing models in biotechnology.

Dark Biotechnology – It refers to applications of biotechnology to weapons and warfare products.

Genetic Engineering

Genetic engineering is an application of biotechnology that involves direct manipulation of an organism's genes. It is a set of technologies used to change the genetic makeup of cells, including the transfer of genes within and across species boundaries to produce improved or novel organisms.

The interest in the phenomena of heredity created the field of genetics, i.e. the study of genes and heredity. In ancient times, people improved plant crops and domesticated animals by selecting desirable individuals for breeding. However, the study of genes as a set of scientific principles and analytical procedures emerged only in the 1860s when the monk Gregor Mendel performed a set of experiments in the monastery garden that revealed the existence of biological "factors" responsible for transmitting traits from generation to generation. These factors were later called genes.

In order to appreciate the extent of developments in the field of genetic engineering, one needs to understand some basic terminologies and processes.

Deoxyribonucleic Acid (DNA)

It is a large biomolecule that contains the complete genetic information for an organism. The basic building block of the DNA is a set of sequences created by four unique nucleotides also known as bases A, G, C and T. This is analogous to how 26 letters of the alphabet can be arranged to create a word. DNA has a helical structure, shaped like a corkscrew. The cell uses DNA as a template to create matching messenger RNA, which controls the process of protein production.

Genes

Each gene is a small segment of DNA that contains a set of instructions for an organism to create a single protein. A single organism may have thousands of genes; and together the entire set of genes is called its genome.

Genes are the functional fundamental units of the heredity; comparable to smallest particle atom in Physics. These are made up of DNA and are passed down from parents to their children. Genes are generally organised and packaged in components called chromosomes. In humans, there are 23 pairs or 46 chromosomes. There are about thirty thousand genes in every cell of the human body.

Proteins

The proteins are probably the most important class of material in the body. Proteins are not just building blocks for muscles, connective tissues, skin, and other structures; they also are needed to make enzymes. Enzymes are complex proteins that control and carry out nearly all chemical processes and reactions within the body. The body produces thousands of different enzymes. The protein synthesis is controlled by genes, which are contained on chromosome

Mutation

A mutation is a change that occurs in the DNA sequence of an organism, either due to mistakes when the DNA is copied, or as the result of environmental factors such as UV light and cigarette smoke. During Pandemic 19, many mutations (Alpha, Bravo, Delta etc.) of SARS Cov-2 virus have emerged.

Gene Editing

Gene editing is a way of making specific changes to the DNA of a cell or organism. An enzyme cuts the DNA at a specific sequence, and when this is repaired by the cell a change or 'edit' is made to the sequence.

Plasmids

A plasmid is a small, extra-chromosomal DNA molecule within a cell that is physically separated from chromosomal DNA and can replicate independently. They are most commonly found as small circular, double-stranded DNA molecules in bacteria. Plasmids have been key to the development of molecular biotechnology. They act as delivery vehicles or vectors to introduce foreign DNA into the bacteria.

Ribonucleic Acid (RNA)

RNA is the acronym for ribonucleic acid. Pieces of RNA are used to construct proteins so that new cell growth may take place. Unlike DNA, the RNA is single-stranded. A central tenet of molecular biology states that the flow of genetic information is from DNA through RNA to proteins.

Gain of Function

It involves deliberately altering an organism by altering a gene or introducing a mutation in a pathogen with a view to enhancing its transmissibility, virulence and immunogenicity. It is done by genetically engineering the virus through a number of iterations and growing them in different mediums.

Genome

The genome of an organism is the entire set of genetic instructions found in a cell. It consists of nucleotide sequences of DNA. Human genome, consisting of 23 pairs of chromosomes and approximately 3.1 billion bases of DNA sequence, has already been mapped.

An international group of scientists is working on the mapping the genetic sequence of SARS C0V-2 virus. This will help trace genetic mutations, re-combination as well as distribution of the virus and also make predictions about the future of its spread.

Virus

Viruses are found in almost every ecosystem on the earth and they form the most numerous type of biological entity. Viruses outnumber bacteria by 10 to 1. The study of viruses is known as virology.

A virus is a small collection of genetic code, either DNA or RNA, surrounded by a protein coat. A virus cannot replicate by itself. Viruses must infect cells and use components of the host cell to make copies of themselves. Because viruses don't have the same components as bacteria, antibiotics cannot kill these. Only antiviral medications or vaccines can eliminate or reduce the severity of viral diseases, including AIDS, COVID-19, measles and smallpox.

CRISPR-Cas9 – A Disruptive Technology

For a long time geneticists used chemicals or radiation to cause mutations. However, they had no way of controlling where in the genome the mutation would occur. So, the techniques lacked precision and predictable outcome. This in turn affected the progress of this field in term of generating applications, as well as, added heavily to the costs of the process.

All this changed dramatically with the arrival in 2013 of a unique CRISPR-Cas9 technology for genome editing. It made the process faster, cheaper and more accurate than previous techniques of editing DNA. This has created immense potential and space for large number of applications.

CRISPR is an acronym for "Clustered Regulatory Interspersed Short Palindromic Repeats". This technology enables geneticists and medical researchers to edit parts of the genome by removing, adding or altering sections of the DNA sequence. It is currently the simplest, most versatile and precise method of genetic manipulation and is therefore causing a buzz in the science world.

The CRISPR-Cas9 system consists of two key molecules that introduce a mutation into the DNA. These are: an enzyme called Cas9 that acts as a pair of 'molecular scissors' that can cut the two strands of DNA at a specific location in the genome so that bits of DNA can then be added or removed. And a piece of RNA called guide RNA binds to DNA and predetermined sequence guides Cas9 to the right part of the genome. The Cas9 makes a cut across both strands of the DNA and then the DNA repair machinery introduces changes to one or more genes

Synthetic Biology

It is a branch of science that encompasses a broad range of methodologies from various disciplines, such as biotechnology, genetic engineering, molecular biology, molecular engineering and systems biology. It is an emerging field that aims to combine the knowledge and methods of biology, engineering and related disciplines in the design of chemically synthesised DNA to create organisms with novel or enhanced characteristics and traits.

There is a need to understand the distinction between the genetic engineering and synthetic biology. The objective of the genetic engineering is simply to modify the genome of an organism or to bring the beneficial traits of one organism to another. On the other hand, synthetic biology seeks to re-engineer entire organisms, create existing organisms using only their genetic base pairs, and even create new ones that have never been seen in nature. Synthetic biology obviously has enormous potential for changing any element of our world—from creating plants that will produce energetic compounds or inexpensive medicines, to producing organisms that neutralise industrial waste.

In synthetic biology, scientists typically stitch together long stretches of DNA and insert them into an organism's genome. These synthesised pieces of DNA could be genes that are found in other organisms or they could be entirely novel. The scientists in the United States synthesised a viral genome for the first time 2002.

While the goals of synthetic biology are beneficial, these capabilities also could be used to cause harm. It should be regarded as dual-use technology. The synthetic biology now affords capabilities to modify or create dangerous microorganisms, including viruses, as evidenced by synthetic development of polio, influenza viruses (and notably the 1918 strain), and horsepox, among others.

Genetics - Transforming Biological Warfare

The genetics has essentially established the modularity of gene structure. These are like building blocks where some of the blocks can be replaced; thereby altering the functionality of the system. Therefore, using the genetic engineering, several techniques are being applied to increase the efficacy of the pathogens for biological warfare. Some of these are:

> Controlled Gene Modification. It involves inserting plasmids, small bacterial DNA fragments, into the DNA of other bacteria in order to increase virulence or other pathogenic properties within the host bacteria. This technique is used for binary bioweapons.

> Designer Genes. With complete genomes available and the aforementioned advances in gene synthesis, scientists will soon be able to design pathogens by creating synthetic genes, synthetic viruses, and possibly entirely new organisms.

> Gene Therapy. Gene therapy involves repairing or replacing a gene of an organism, permanently changing its genetic composition. By replacing existing genes with harmful genes, this technique can be used to manufacture biological weapons.

> Stealth Viruses. An interesting technique, the stealth viruses are viral infections that enter the cells and remain dormant for an extended amount of time until triggered externally to cause the disease. In the context of warfare, these viruses could be spread to a large population, and activation could either be delayed or used as a threat for blackmail.

> Host-Swapping. As with Ebola virus, the animal viruses could be genetically modified and developed to infect humans. This could act as a potent bioweapon.

> Genome Seeker. It involves designing a pathogen that targets a specific person's genome. This agent may spread through

populations showing minimal or no symptoms, yet it would be fatal to the intended target. It would enable targeting of a specific ethnicity.

Smart Biological Weapons

In the past thirty years, the biotechnology has been revolutionised by molecular biology and genetic engineering. These techniques evolved, for control of infectious diseases and vaccine development can also be used to create deadlier biological weapons.

The gene-editing techniques such as CRISPR could lead to development of novel or modified pathogens that would spread quickly, infect larger number of people, cause sickness of greater severity or resist treatment. Viruses and bacteria could be genetically engineered to evade the human immune system.

 Another area of concern is the development of pathogens for carrying out targeted assassinations. It is quite feasible to edit the genes of a deadly virus so that it would affect only a single target based on his or her genetic code.

The stealth viruses are another area of interest. These viral infections enter the cells and remain dormant for an extended period until triggered externally to cause the disease. This could enable the use of bioweapons in a clandestine manner.

In the foreseeable future, there are likely to be biological weapons with small footprint to be used at a specific time and place of attacker's choosing with defined parameters of nature and scale of devastation. Viruses modified through genetic engineering may become the preferred option as weapons of mass destruction. A term has been coined for such a weapon – "Virus – the Braham Astra". Time will test the veracity of this nomination.

Another likelihood is that advances in gene editing could allow scientists to develop biological weapons capable of discriminating among target populations based on ethnic, racial, or other genetically defined characteristics. Such biological weapon systems may be the result of convergence of many technologies like Artificial Intelligence, mathematical modeling and computers.

Accessibility of Biological Weapons

The genetic engineering has influenced the development of biological weapons in many ways. Lower cost of technology has made the access relatively easier. Further, the biological weapons themselves will become more potent. These factors will make these weapons attractive to rogue states and non-state actors. Further, the dual- use nature of the technology allows weapon development programs to continue in secrecy.

Therefore, global efforts to limit the proliferation of biological weapons face many challenges. Easier access may lead to many states acquiring biological weapons. Topping this would be the dual –use aspect of the life sciences making the verification process more tedious.

Virulence and Transmissibility – Changes in Viral Genome

Often, it is the small variances in the viral genome that can cause a difference in its virulence and transmissibility. Changes to the viral genome can be caused by an antigenic shift where two viruses can combine to form a new viral subtype.

An antigenic shift can be caused by mutations resulting from errors that occur during the process of viral replication. Different variants of SARS CoV-2 virus that have appeared at different points of time belong to this category, including the Delta variant. As is well known, the level of transmissibility and the severity of disease caused by these variants vary.

1918 Influenza Virus

The influenza pandemic of 1918–20 following World War I was quite severe causing an estimated 50 million deaths worldwide. As the microbiological science was not understood at that time, the viral that caused the pandemic could not be analysed. People observed some rudimentary precautions to ward off the disease.

However, the scientists through reverse genetics have been able to reconstruct the virus that caused Spanish flu. The reconstructed virus has exhibited very severe virulence. Naturally, its correlation with

SARS CoV-2 virus is being studied with relation to their origin and evolutionary process.

Pandemic 19 – Is Virus Genetically Engineered?

As part of the debate on the origin of SARS CoV-2 virus, the scientific community and intelligence agencies are quite divided in their opinions. One of the theories being considered is that the virus was intentionally engineered and that its escape resulted from a laboratory leak at the Wuhan Institute of Virology in China.

Given the Chinese capabilities in the field of genetic engineering, it is quite feasible to intentionally engineer a virus that could cause Covid-19 pandemic. However, SARS CoV-2 virus does not appear to be built around the backbone of any known virus. Therefore, the probability of the virus having been engineered in the Wuhan laboratory may be low, but cannot be discounted.

At the same time, China has been less than forthcoming in permitting a thorough scientific investigation in the matter. This reluctance on part of the Chinese authorities adds fuel to speculative theories. It is important to trace the origin of the virus, as it is an essential part of preparedness to fight future pandemics.

Even if genetic engineering wasn't behind the current pandemic, it could very well unleash the next one. The heavy disruption caused in global economic systems exemplifies the devastation potential that bioengineered virus hold. The state and non-state actors will definitely be evaluating the use of such biological weapons to achieve their aim.

Genetic Data Collection by China

Based on American Intelligence agencies reports, it has been stated in the print media on October 24, 2021 that the Chinese firms are collecting genetic data from around the world. It is part of an effort by the Chinese government and the companies to develop the world's largest bio-database. China intends to dominate the field of biotechnology and is using legal and illegal means to acquire the necessary know how.

These intelligence agencies have stressed the intersection of different technologies and genetic and biological research as an area of competition and espionage. They further mention that the Chinese government is collecting medical, health and genetic data around the world so that it has an edge on developing cures for future pandemics. An earlier report stated that China uses genetic tests to track members of the Uighurs, a predominant Muslim minority group. A Chinese company is reported to have developed a neonatal genetic test in conjunction with Chinese military that has enabled them to collect genetic data of millions of people around the world.

Two things stand out from the above reports. First, China foresees a great potential in genetics and molecular sciences; and it desires to dominate the world in this area. Second, the Chinese military is actively involved in various projects related to genetics and molecular sciences. This has a direct bearing on the development of future genetically engineered biological weapons and global security.

Take Aways

The ongoing revolution in biotechnology has transformed the biological warfare in many ways. With future generations of CRISPR-like technology and an advances in molecular sciences, there would be no theoretical end to the misery that could be caused.

Recent developments in genetics like gain of function technology, gene editing and synthetic biology are having a deep impact on conceptualising and developing new set of biological weapons. The range of biological weapons now spans binary weapons, stealth weapons and weapons with special identification characteristics. CRISPR technology has provided the scientists with a versatile tool to carry out gene editing and manipulation at fraction of a cost incurred in the past.

With easy accessibility, many players other than major powers would be attracted into undertaking development of biological weapons. New strategies may have to be devised to tackle the challenges of proliferation. It can be said that the genetic engineering has ushered in "New Age Biological Warfare"

Strategic Thought – *Military Imperatives*

Before delving deep into this subject, it is important to clarify some doubts that arise often like: is the biological warfare likely at all; being a signatory to Biological and Toxin Weapons Conference, 1972 (BTWC) India does not subscribe to the idea of biological weapons; use of biological weapons endangers own troops because of blow back, it is a dirty weapon; the treaty will ensure no one owns and uses a biological weapon etc. Because of such apprehensions, the study and preparedness to fight against a biological attack have been relegated to low down the order. An examination of the issue is therefore called for.

> *"Victory at all costs, victory in spite of all terror, victory however long and hard the road may be; for without victory, there is no survival"*
>
> *- Winston Churchill*

The above maxim would be applicable to any country engaged in a war. If the advances in technology make available a weapon which gives decided advantage over the adversary, it will surely find its way into one's arsenal. Ongoing revolution in Biotechnology has transformed the lethality and transmissibility of biological weapons to an extent that these can break the back of even major powers. So, don't expect a country to shun a Braham Astra (virus-based Biological Weapon) if it has access to one.

Believing that the BTWC treaty would ensure that no one would develop and acquire such weapons may prove costly. In the absence of a verification mechanism, this treaty is weak and lacks compliance. It has been flagrantly violated in the past. If the treaty enjoyed everyone's confidence, why would there be persistent suggestions that SARS CoV-2 virus is a Chinese biological weapon that got released accidentally.

The treaties and international laws are one thing — and humanity's ability to find novel ways of killing each other is another.

It is known that the effects of biological weapons are difficult to control or to predict in a battlefield situation due to the blowback phenomenon. This entails risk to own troops. The concern is justified as of today, but synthetic biology is generating options to overcome the problem.

Finally, the spectrum of warfare is generally restricted to strategic, operational and tactical spheres. It overlooks other security threats like bioterrorism. The realisation that in 2001 a handful of envelopes containing anthrax were sufficient to cause widespread panic in the US is a clear demonstration of the power of cheap biological weapons. Relatively cheap to produce and with disproportionately large effect, biological weapons make themselves a strong candidate for use by the terrorists and in asymmetric warfare. BTWC, 1972 is not in a position to dissuade terrorist outfits from acquiring biological weapons.

Therefore, the biological weapons pose a real security threat, which cannot be ignored. It must form part of the security matrix so that rightful focus is maintained on biosecurity and preparedness to protect own troops against a biological strike. Also, at the national level, sufficient resources should be deployed for advanced research in genetics and molecular sciences.

At Russian military college, there has been a gradual priority shift within the Nuclear, Chemical and Biological (NBC) triad as far as time devoted to different subjects is concerned. While previously nuclear element was the most important element of the triad, followed by chemical and biological elements, it is the biological element that has replaced the nuclear one to become Number One in the NBC triad. Adequate appreciation of these non-conventional threats is essential so that sufficient resources are deployed towards development of doctrines and operational concepts, training and preparedness.

Strategic Thought

Post World War II, during the Cold War period; there was a rush to acquire nuclear weapons. With then Soviet Union on one side and the USA and its allies on the other, the type, size and the numbers of nuclear weapons were used to define the super power status. Doctrines like Mutually Assured Destruction (MAD) aptly described the future of mankind. Eventually, through a number of treaties and regulatory framework, a semblance of stability was achieved in the development and deployment of nuclear weapons. These became the means of deterrence.

The break up of Soviet Union brought about major global geo-political changes with the USA emerging as the sole superpower. Then began the dominance of the battlefield by the advanced technologies. The battlefield was transformed into a multi-dimensional space with the use of long range missile, satellites, electromagnetic radiation, cyber attacks, precision-guided ammunition, autonomous systems and over the horizon technologies. This led to development of new technology led concepts and the physical combat moved lower down the order. Modern military thought found reflection in terms like: shock and awe, fire and fury, fire from the sky, network centric war and manoeuvre warfare etc.

In this breathtaking battlefield scenario, the biological warfare seemed unglamorous. It receded, to the extent of exclusion, from the minds of the strategic planners. However, all this changed in 2019 when the world was hit by the SARS CoV- 2 virus.

Covid -19 Pandemic is the closest one can get to experience Biological Warfare. While, the pandemic has been treated as a civil catastrophe, it has all the makings of a military operation. The scale and speed of the spread of the pathogen has conjured up the images of use of nuclear weapons in the minds of the strategic community.

Being the weapons of mass destruction, it would be natural to consider various strategic concepts and doctrines pertaining to the use of biological weapons as analogous to nuclear weapons. It is during the cold war that the concepts like nuclear deterrence, no first use, non-proliferation and nuclear umbrella were enunciated. The relevance of such concepts to Biological Warfare needs to be examined, as well as there is need to consider new operational imperatives that have emerged.

Spectrum of Biological Warfare

Biological warfare has been part of non-conventional warfare from early times. Also known as germ warfare, it used disease as a weapon to defeat the enemy. The recent technological and microbiological advances enabled the development of true biological weapons, some of which were used as in the case of the Japanese during World War II.

The spectrum of potential biological hazards is very wide. It is the deliberate use of living organisms to cause disease in humans, animals or plants as an act of war. The biological weapons can be employed at strategic, operational and tactical levels. Their deployment is guided by factors like high potency, low visibility, relative ease of delivery, capacity to cause mass casualties and the time lag involved due to incubation period.

Apart from making the battlefield non-linear, biological weapons have expanded the vastness of battle space. The boundaries between the borders, frontiers and the hinterland have been diffused. The active domain of biological warfare may encompass both combatants as well as civilians.

Further, it includes the battles of the grey zone – asymmetric, bioterrorism, unrestricted warfare etc. The advances in synthetic biology promise customised biological weapons, which would suit the contemplated nature of task.

In addition to the above, even fighting a pandemic may bear the stamp of a military operation. Most of the planning and resources built for bio defence can always be gainfully employed during biological emergencies anywhere in the country. This aspect was highlighted during the fight against Covid-19.

Strategic Concepts

There is currently very limited literature that expounds on the strategic doctrines for biological warfare. Renowned military scholars have not delved into this subject simply because biological weapons have not played any prominent role in any of the major wars.

However, as the theme of this book suggests, the revolution in biotechnology holds promise of developing biological agents with much greater lethality, infectivity and transmissibility. Therefore, the use of highly potent biological weapons for causing mass devastation in a future conflict is a distinct possibility and there is a dire need to evolve strategic concepts and doctrines for the biological warfare.

This is a preliminary effort to enunciate some biological warfare strategic concepts based on two guiding factors. First, the genetic engineering has enabled mapping of the genome and CRISPR technology has provided the tools to manipulate structure of a virus to produce future Braham Astras. Second, much of the strategic thought has been borrowed from Nuclear Weapons in an analogous manner as both belong to the WMD category.

Deterrence

The biological weapons are often compared with nuclear weapons in terms of the destruction that they cause. Under the right conditions, a biological attack could kill as many people as a nuclear device. This similarity is the basis for most analyses that suggest that biological weapons will have similar political effects as nuclear weapons. However, this issue requires deeper examination.

The pre-requisite for strategic deterrence is the capability of the one targeted to retaliate by inflicting unacceptable damage against its attacker. During the cold war, the possession of nuclear weapons by both super-powers gave rise to the situation of mutual deterrence described as mutual assured destruction (MAD). It is a doctrine of military strategy and national security policy in which a full-scale use of nuclear weapons by two or more opposing sides would cause the complete annihilation of both the attacker and defender.

Although the biological weapons have the potential to inflict unacceptable damage against an adversary, these are different from nuclear weapons in many ways. First, there is considerable time delay from the time the biological weapon is launched to the time it is detected by those under attack. Any retaliation with a biological weapon will further add to the time element; thus allowing the attacker time to gear up its defences. Second, unlike for the nuclear attack, some defensive countermeasures are feasible against a biological attack, which mitigate the fear of retaliation. It can therefore be inferred that the deterrence built into the classical MAD concept will not work in case of biological warfare.

Yet, it is felt that deterrence can be achieved by displaying the will to use overwhelming retaliatory force in other domains to inflict unacceptable damage on the attacker. This could be referred to as the Retaliatory Assured Destruction (RAD). This may involve the threat of nuclear strike or powerful conventional weapons attack against the perpetrator state. Therefore, RAD stated in clear terms will deter any state planning to use biological weapons. The Americans have strategic commitment to launch a nuclear counterstrike to discourage a biological weapons attack against the United States.

Offensive Deployment

Biological weapons are primarily offensive in nature. The offence – defence balance in biological warfare strongly favours the attacker because developing and using biological weapon to cause casualties is significantly easier and less expensive than developing and fielding defences against them. Whether the biotechnology revolution will strengthen the defender or allow attackers to maintain their edge in this competition is unknown. Four factors help to determine the attacker's advantage in biological warfare: the potency of biological weapons, the diversity of threat agents, the ease of surprise and the difficulty in defending against such an attack.

The biological weapons may be employed in various ways to gain strategic advantage on the enemy. These may shape the battlefield to deny the enemy freedom of action and break its coherence. The aim is to curtail the enemy's combat power and create vulnerabilities in its core areas.

The erstwhile Soviet Union's military doctrine for use of biological weapons contained two contingencies: strategic and operational use. The primary use contemplated would be strategic—that is, large-scale deployment of biological weapons against strategic targets in an enemy state during the course of a "total war." This strategic-use doctrine focused on counter-value targeting of cities and civilian populations.

The Soviet Union developed this doctrine specifically vis-à-vis the United States and reportedly planned for the use of biological weapons parallel to nuclear weapons.

The second contingency of the operational use, contemplated deploying biological weapons against deep military targets on the battlefield, around 100 to 150 kilometers beyond the front lines. The focus on deep targets was envisaged because the biological weapons could have highly unpredictable effects, including the possible infection of one's own military forces.

Asymmetric Strategy

It is the strategy to fight an asymmetric war, i.e. war between the unequal. The word asymmetric refers to the significant disparity in size of forces, advanced weaponry, the strength of economy etc., between the two opponents.

Such huge disparities provide weak state or non-state actors with strong incentives to employ biological weapons as part of an asymmetric strategy that may outweigh the political or strategic imperatives. The relatively low cost of acquisition and easy accessibility of biological weapons makes these a weapon of choice for the weaker side. Their capacity to cause massive devastation and produce tremendous psychological impact add to their attractiveness.

It is expected that the impending advances in biotechnology are likely to play a major role in future asymmetric warfare.

Unrestrained War – Multi-dimensional Battle Space

Lately, the Chinese military scholars have propounded a concept of "Unrestricted Warfare". This form of warfare follows no rules, knows no boundaries between military forces and civilian population, does not recognise international norms and bears no taboos. It propagates all such measures, which weaken the opponent's resolve and capacity to fight a war.

It proposes that the battle encompasses local, regional, national and international spaces. It aims at seeking out opponent's vulnerabilities and then striking these. Through surprise, the opponent is to be caught off guard and unprepared to defend itself. It is in line with Sun Tzu's maxim "The supreme art of war is to subdue the enemy without fighting."

To a discernable military strategist, all the above propositions suggest undertaking successful biological warfare operations. Given the Chinese propensity towards conducting advanced biological research in various laboratories like Wuhan Institute of Virology, the basic strategy of unrestricted warfare is closely linked to the use of biological weapons.

Biological Umbrella

The United States has used nuclear weapons to "extend deterrence" and shield some of its allies from early in the nuclear age. It has gone to considerable lengths to make its nuclear umbrella credible; partly to discourage enemies from attacking but also to convince its allies not to get nuclear weapons themselves. This concept of providing nuclear umbrella was to promote nuclear non-proliferation.

Like the concept of nuclear umbrella, a global concept of biological umbrella may have to be evolved, so that the smaller powers/countries can be weaned away from pursuing biological weapon programs. Some, similar protection may be needed against bioterrorism. This could be one of the steps in promoting non-proliferation of biological weapons.

Small Footprint - Big Bang

Biological weapons have a small footprint: with no blast or boom, they do not require elaborate launch pads and safe silos. Also, they can be launched in small quantities from dispersed locations.

At the strategic level of warfare, the goal is to reduce the willingness or ability of the enemy to continue to prosecute a war. States can achieve this objective either through attacks targeted at civilians, with the goal of increasing pressure on the government to yield, or through attacks aimed at damaging the enemy's economy to the point where the state can no longer effectively resist.

Biological warfare can target civilians directly with anti-personal agents or indirectly with anti-livestock or anti-crop agents that could be used against agricultural targets to reduce an enemy's food supply. The delayed effects of biological weapons and uncertainties surrounding travel of aerosol cloud are less important for strategic attacks that do not require precision or immediate results. In addition, the disproportionate fear that these dreaded weapons evoke could amplify the psychological impact of even a small-scale biological weapon attack.

Fog of Ambiguities and Uncertainties

National security gets greatly weakened in case there is an environment of ambiguities and uncertainties pertaining to a security threat. This is exactly what can be achieved by employing a suitable biological weapon.

Consider various features of biological weapons like: odourless, colourless, silent, act with a time delay, cause sickness and quickly spread to other areas in a non-linear manner. Moreover, this weapon can be transported in an innocuous manner and released clandestinely. Long after, when the biological attack is identified by the state, it is extremely difficult to pinpoint the source of origin or to get hold of those who have carried out the attack. Therefore, the state is unable to hold anyone to account or to initiate punitive measures. On the whole, the nation gets enveloped in a fog of ambiguities and uncertainties, which can be further exploited by an opponent through the psychological warfare. This is a very effective offensive strategy.

Command and Control

Being weapons of mass destruction with strategic impact, the command and control on employment of biological weapons must be vested in strategic command, as in the case of nuclear weapons. In time to come, more sophisticated delivery systems would be available, yet small special forces groups will continue to play an important role in deployment of biological weapons. It is visualised that while the planning and control may be exercised centrally at the level of strategic command, the execution would have to be delegated to respective theatre commands.

Another major difference in the deployment of biological weapons would be that some top public health professionals would have to be taken into confidence to ensure the safety of own civilian population.

Agriculture and Animal Husbandry

Food security is an integral part of national security. The former can be adversely impacted through the release of anti-crop biological agents, which may be attempted by bioterrorists or in a state-to-state conflict.

The vulnerability in the field of agriculture has increased due to recent scientific research in genetically modified crops. This grand effort to increase the yield from the limited availability of land has a flip side. While genetic engineering opens the way for bountiful crops, it is equally capable of producing genetically modified weeds and anti-crop agents. It is an important concern requiring deliberations under the aegis of ministry of agriculture.

The use of a biological weapon on livestock could have a serious detrimental effect on a country's supply chain. It could result in the loss of valuable animals, costs related to the containment of outbreaks and the disposal of carcasses, loss of trade and other economic effects. It must be remembered that the animals are much less guarded as compared to the human targets; thus their vulnerability to the introduction of biological agents is high.

Operational Imperatives

The military Commanders in the field would be required to oversee the employment of biological weapons against the enemy as well as ensure various bio defence measures. While undertaking biological attack, the Commander would aim to substantially downgrade the enemy's combat potential by inflicting casualties among their soldiers, causing breakdown of chain of command and disrupting the logistic chain. On the other hand, defending against a likely biological attack would entail elaborate surveillance measures, casualty management and evacuation, protective gear and decontamination tools.

Omni - Space Battlefield

This particular term is being used for the first time to define biological warfare battlefield. So far, the general term being used is that " battlefield is everywhere", which refers to the physical extent of the battle spaces. Omni-space battlefield, not only refers to physical extent, but also covers domains like healthcare, economy, industry and trade, social life etc. For biological warfare, the term Omni-space battlefield is therefore considered more versatile.

The above description of the battlefield is highly important when it comes to carrying out strategic planning for biodefence. It is no longer a fight by the defence forces alone, but the combined potential of all non-defence agencies coupled with the defence forces that have to be brought to bear on the battlefield.

As part of the national bio strategy, synergistic systems must be developed to harness the potential of military and civil enterprises. There has to be unity of command and at the same time sharing of information and resources in an uninhibited manner. Various distinctions will need to be blurred to ensure coordinated functioning. It should truly depict " a nation goes to war".

Theatre and Tactical Level Biological Weapons

The military value of biological weapons lies in the characteristics of the type of weapon deployed and the doctrines adopted. The diversity of biological agents available provides multiple options on the type of missions to be undertaken against a range of targets. These weapons have limited utility at the tactical level due to delayed effects of the biological agents and the lack of precision attached to the aerosol clouds. Yet, the aerosol clouds enable penetration of bunkers and buildings, which may be difficult to penetrate otherwise.

Biological weapons may have the greatest military utility at the operational or theatre level of warfare. The goal of attacks on logistical networks, reinforcements and command and control facilities would be to introduce operational paralysis, which reduces the enemy's ability to move and coordinate forces in the theatre. The ability of some biological weapons to sicken victims for weeks or months could also outweigh the delayed effects of such agents. The power projection forces that rely on a small number of large facilities with primarily civilian workforces are particularly vulnerable to such disruptive attacks. As a result, the employment of biological weapons against theatre targets could serve as a potent force multiplier for a conventional military operation.

Technologically strong militaries have come to rely greatly on air power and seaborne flotillas to project their power; thereby reducing the number of combat troops involved in the fighting. Corollary to this situation is that their airbases or major warships present themselves as highly valuable targets for biological attacks. Few incidents can be mentioned in this regard. North Korea has contemplated biological weapons attacks on US airbases with a view to bringing down their air superiority as well as to cause fear and panic. Other instance pertains to the aircraft carrier HMS Queen Elizabeth, the newest flagship and pride of the Royal Navy, reporting nearly 100 cases of Covid 19 aboard the vessel during July 2021. The strike group was on a global tour, and impact of the outbreak on the mission has not been made public for obvious reasons.

In another case, Type 23 frigate HMS Northumberland was forced to return to Devonport Naval Base in December 2020 on the outbreak of Covid 19 aboard the vessel. While, these incidents pertain to natural occurrence of the disease, but it equally well illustrates the huge impact a deliberately engineered biological attack could have on the operational capabilities of a large naval force.

Threat Assessment – Bio Defence

Accurate and timely intelligence has long been regarded as a crucial element in defending against biological weapons strikes. Strict secrecy and the dual-use nature of biotechnology make biological weapons programs a difficult target to track for intelligence agencies. Bio threat assessments must take into account not only the capabilities that are challenging to monitor but also the intentions that are even more difficult to discern. In fact, the most significant intelligence breakthroughs have resulted from defections by insiders. Only such insiders can provide the information on the intent that is required for a comprehensive understanding of a state's biological warfare program.

The threat posed by terrorists is likely to be even more difficult given the intensive secretive nature of such organisations. A terrorist group with the motivation and capability to use these weapons may emerge with little or no warning.

The history is replete with examples of flawed bio threat assessments that were either overestimates or underestimates of an adversary's biological warfare capabilities and intentions. During World War II, the US military grossly underestimated the Japanese biological warfare program until it was able to interview personnel captured during and after the war. During the Cold War, the United States and its allies lacked a clear understanding of the Soviet biological weapons program.

Bio Defence Measures - Operational and Tactical Levels

Future threat environment should take into account the likely use of biological weapons by a potential adversary. Accordingly, bio defence measures should be planned and implemented to counter any such challenge to security.

An effective step would be to strengthen defence against most threatening agents through improved detection, diagnosis, therapy and vaccines. This would create doubts about the chances of success in the mind of the attacker and who may then desist from using a biological weapon. At the same time, the access to biological weapons should be made difficult through various control measures.

Preparedness and Protection

Early detection of and response to biological strike is crucial. Without special preparation at various levels, a large-scale attack with a biological agent could cause large number of casualties and overwhelm the medical support infrastructure in the field.

Usually, military forces have a certain degree of preparedness in place to meet the challenges of a biological attack on the front line. They create a surveillance network based on biosensors; establish pathogen analysis facilities in field hospitals and communication system to notify troops in the vicinity about a bio-attack so that preventive measures can be immediately initiated. There is a proper system for treating and evacuation of sick persons. To maintain uniformity of action across board, detailed standard operating procedures (SOPs) are issued.

This template with due modifications can be adopted by the civil authorities. In any case, a close liaison between military and civil authorities is essential to tackle all challenges posed by a bio strike along the border or a bioterrorist attack in the interior or the occurrence of a pandemic.

There are many protective measures that can be undertaken at the individual and unit level. These must be adopted early enough so as to minimise the damage. Different protective measures include protective clothing, masks, goggles etc. The decontamination kit should be in place for ready use if required.

Intelligence

The intelligence about the enemy's biological weapons capability can be most helpful in countering such threat. The knowledge about the specific agents being developed or manufactured can guide the vaccine efforts, creating appropriate detection methodologies and for gearing up the medical infrastructure.

While major part of intelligence input will emanate from the national and higher headquarters levels, local information may be used to refine the inferences. Technical and tactical intelligence about an impending biological strike can be of immense value in neutralising its adverse effect. Sufficient resources must be deployed to garner such intelligence.

Detection and Surveillance

The detection is undertaken by putting up biosensors in different locations. These sensors are able to detect and identify different pathogens, which may be present in the environment. These are deployed in the form of a grid and connected to a control station. They raise an immediate alarm in case of a biological agent strike. Biosensor technology has seen much advancement with the sensitivity of detection having improved considerably.

On the other hand, the surveillance calls for close monitoring of unusual sickness among the troops and taking steps to get the disease diagnosed at the earliest. Any such case must be reported upwards, where the information can be collated and the pattern of the spread of disease can be established. If the presence of any infectious disease is discerned, all actions as per SOP get into motion.

Digital Technologies and Communications

One of the outstanding features of the fight against ongoing pandemic Covid-19 has been the exploitation of digital technologies and communication systems in controlling the spread of disease. Based on this experience, the military will do well to upgrade its own systems.

The availability of these technologies facilitates decision making at different levels and thus cut down on the response times. Various artificial intelligence tools enable accurate diagnosis and suggest therapies and protocols for treating patients.

Reliable communications are an essential requirement for detectors, surveillance systems, computers and data devices. In the remote areas, special attention has to be paid to making available stable power supply.

Vaccination

If the biological threat is established in advance through intelligence or other sources, an effective protective measure is to vaccinate the troops in the vicinity of likely area of strike. Immunisation can mitigate the adverse effects of a biological agent. However, it requires close coordination between the national public health authorities, virology research laboratories and defence medical authorities. It is not a on the spot activity, but part of ongoing preparatory efforts.

Currently, there are licensed vaccines available for a few threats, such as anthrax and smallpox, and research is underway to develop and produce vaccines for other threats, such as tularemia, Ebola virus, and Marburg virus. Many biological weapon disease threats, however, lack a corresponding vaccine and this is work in progress.

Also, there is flip side to vaccinating the troops, it can cause stress among those not vaccinated. It is, therefore, essential to educate the troops about the appropriate protective measures and to keep everyone well informed.

Training

Like in any other form of warfare, proper training curricula have to be drawn out for all levels of command. At the level of troops, various drills should be regularly rehearsed. Apart from efficiently sailing through a contingency, practicing different roles raises the psychological confidence of troops about functioning in a difficult environment.

Since multiple agencies would be involved in facing biological emergency, the training must be oriented towards generating greater coordination and continuously revising and refining the guidelines.

Medical Preparedness

Medical infrastructure in a combat zone should be capable of responding to a biological emergency. There is every possibility that all available resources will get overstretched: yet small amount of reserve must be held to supplement effort at the point of criticality. Also, the adequacy of medical response can be greatly enhanced through initial preparedness. A comprehensive standard operating procedure can be of great help for ensuring smooth and quick handling of casualties as well as optimal utilisation of resources.

Different protocols for diagnosis and management of patients suspected of being subjected to a biological attack should be disseminated within the medical echelons. If medical experts cannot be available in-situ, telemedicine facilities may be considered.

The Last Word

Warfare is a constantly evolving enterprise. Advancements in technology keep transforming the combat environment. It is always an endeavour of the armed forces to develop doctrines, concepts and tactics in keeping with the changing environment.

While the research in offensive use of biological agents has been banned under the charter of BTWC 1972, certain countries are undertaking research in biological weapons disguised under cover of dual-use technology. They pose a threat of biological warfare in future, which must not be ignored.

Bioterrorism – *An Asymmetric Power Play*

A handful of envelopes containing B. *anthracis* in 2001 caused widespread panic and precipitated the first evacuation of the houses of the US government since the war of 1812. This clearly demonstrated the power of cheap biological weapons, which are perfectly suited for asymmetric warfare. With their disproportionately strong effect on targeted populations, the biological weapons hold high attraction for terrorists and fringe groups.

Terrorism, in its broadest sense, is the unlawful use of intentional violence to achieve political aims. The terrorism as a means to an end is generally a tactics of the weaker side in an asymmetric conflict. It primarily involves the use of violence against civilians during peacetime. Normally, the terrorists employ conventional weapons; however, when they use biological weapons, their acts are referred to as bioterrorism.

Today, terrorist groups who seek to inflict massive casualties are more loosely organised, espouse an ideology that transcends national borders. They seek to kill infidels and to establish their own caliphates. Such organisations are harder to penetrate and raise a greater sense of concern about the likelihood of their use of a weapon of mass destruction to achieve their objective to inflict mass casualties. They possess the human, material and financial resources to acquire biological weapons and carry the inclination to employ bioterrorism.

A bioterrorism attack is classified as the deliberate release of a pathogen – viral, bacterial, toxin etc – with the intention of causing harm to a human, animal, plant or other living organisms in order to influence government or to intimidate civilian population. Often these are pathogens that occur naturally, but in future they could be subject to gain-of-function processor or other novel features to increase transmissibility and pathogenicity.

The likely scenarios of bioterrorism may include the use of psychotic substances to contaminate food; the use of toxins and poisons in political assassinations, raids with crude biological cloud bombs; the use of dried viral preparations in spray powders; and low flying cruise missiles to dispense genetically-engineered micro-organisms. Much improvisation and innovation is possible in choosing the place and manner of a biological attack.

While biological warfare aims at killing soldiers in the field, bioterrorism is perpetrated on the civilians with the goal of causing disruption in society. The soldiers are provided protective gear to safeguard them against a biological attack. However, the civilian population is more vulnerable to acts of bioterrorism.

Asymmetric Warfare

In the last few decades, a perceptible shift is becoming apparent in the nature of warfare. Big powers are not seeking to fight long, drawn-out wars with huge armies lined up on either side. Traditional large military operations are becoming smaller, faster and asymmetric. Complex operations other than war are gaining favour.

The asymmetric warfare involves the adoption of unconventional strategies and tactics by a force when the military capabilities of belligerent powers are unequal and significantly different. This precludes any direct action by the weaker party. Under these circumstances, the biological weapons become an attractive option for the weaker side. Of late, asymmetric warfare is becoming a chosen means of conflict resolution, even for major powers. A likely example of this in future could be China using hybrid warfare to gain control of Taiwan.

Biological weapons in the hands of the weaker force confer upon it the capability to cause mass casualties and economic damage. A small quantity of biological agent is enough to cause harmful effects. Lately, Covid-19 pandemic has exposed the vulnerability of the world to the use of biological weapons by a rogue state or a terrorist group.

Incidents of Bioterrorism

Through the ages, disgruntled elements of the population with ethnic, nationalistic and ideological grievances have undertaken bioterrorism. These attacks aimed for limited casualties. However, extremist religious terror groups such as al-Qaeda and Japan's Aum Shinrikyo have shown a proclivity for highly lethal attacks. Some incidents of covert assassinations and bioterrorism in the recent times are narrated below.

In 1978 a Bulgarian exile named Georgi Markov was attacked and killed in London. This assassination later became known as the "umbrella killing," because the weapon used was a device disguised as an umbrella. This weapon discharged a tiny pellet into Markov's leg while he was waiting at a bus stop in London. The following day, he became severely ill, and died three days after the attack. It was revealed in later years, this assassination was carried out by the communist Bulgarian secret service, and the technology to commit the crime was supplied to the Bulgarians by the Soviet Union. The pallet was made from an exotic alloy of iridium and platinum and contained the toxin ricin.

In the USA, the much-publicised case is that of the deliberate contamination of salad bars in 1984, with Salmonella typhimurium, an intestinal pathogen. The bioterrorist act, carried out by members of the Rajnishee cult in Oregon, was aimed at securing an electoral result by incapacitating voters. A total of 751 cases of severe enteritis were reported. Though the origin of the epidemic could not be conclusively identified, a member of the cult in 1986 confirmed that it was a deliberate biological attack.

In the mid-1990s, large amounts of botulinum toxin were found in a laboratory in a safe house of the Red Army Faction in Paris, France. Apparently, the toxin was never used.

In Japan, Aum Shinrikyo cult released the nerve agent sarin in a Tokyo subway in 1995 following failure to obtain the Ebola virus for weaponisation in 1992 from (then) Zaire. They also made a failed attempt to release anthrax spores from a building and botulinum toxin from a vehicle.

During Operation Desert Storm, the USA and the coalition of allied countries faced the threat of biological and chemical warfare from Iraq. It was a classic case of asymmetric warfare, where a weak state was taking on a superpower and its allies. However, no biological weapons were used by Iraq during this conflict, possibly fearing a strong retaliation by the USA.

One week after the September 11 terrorist attack on twin towers in the USA, the country was rocked by anthrax attacks beginning September 18, 2001. Letters containing anthrax spores were mailed to several news media offices and to Democrat Senators. It killed five people and infected 17 others. A major FBI investigation followed and finally the suspect was identified as Bruce Ivins, a scientist at the government biodefense laboratory. However, the individual committed suicide before he could be charged with the crime.

A 29 years old Tunisian man in Germany was charged in 2018 with producing a biological weapon. The police during a search of his apartment in the city of Cologne found highly toxic ricin.

He came to Germany in 2016 and had sympathies towards the Islamic State. The security services first became suspicious after he ordered 1,000 castor seeds – the main ingredient for producing ricin – and a coffee grinder from an online store.

Above incidents are only the reported ones, while there would have been many unsuccessful attempts that have passed unnoticed. Point to note is that there has been a close connection between the terrorists and the biological weapons and it is likely to continue in future as well.

Suitability of Biological Weapons for Terrorists

Biological weapons possess certain special features that make them attractive for the terrorists. Biological agents are difficult to detect, economical and easy to use, thus making them appealing to the terrorists. Also, the time delay involved in incubation of the disease, allows the operators of covert operation to make good their escape. The cost of production of these WMDs is manageable and this effort can be disguised as a biotechnology venture for commercial purposes.

Anonymity

The biological weapons are relatively easy to develop in secrecy and are well suited for covert delivery. Since, there is considerable time delay between the release of biological agent and its effects being detected through sick people or otherwise, it allows the perpetrators to escape from the scene incognito.

Accessibility of Technology

Unlike the nuclear weapon technology, the field of biotechnology requires limited investments of financial and human resources. Being a dual use technology, the equipment and know how can be acquired through legitimate channels. Much knowledge of this technology can be attained through open source domains on the Internet and through published literature.

Delivery and Dissemination

Only a small amount of biological agent has to be delivered to the site. A small special action team can transport it in an innocuous manner. Since, these are odourless and colourless, the chances of their detection are remote. No intricate delivery means are required. As regards the dissemination of the agent, it could be done through contact, using the wind or spreading them from high buildings, crop sprayers, commercial aircraft, and helicopters. The contamination of food and water supplies could be another significant mode of dissemination.

Fear and Panic

The biological weapons are unique in their invisibility and their delayed effects. These factors generate fear and cause confusion among the victims and other state agencies. A biological warfare attack would not only cause sickness and death in a large number of victims but would also aim to create fear, panic, and paralysing uncertainty. Its goal is disruption of social and economic activity, and the breakdown of government authority.

Mass Devastation

Their capacity to cause mass devastation makes biological weapons a powerful tool in the hands of terrorists. The threat of their use may enable the non-state actors to gain an upper hand during the negotiations. Post the devastation caused by Covid-19 pandemic, the value of this currency (possession of biological weapons) has gone up many fold.

Choice of Biological Agents

There are numerous potential biological agents. The choice of the biowarfare agent depends on the economic, technical, and financial capabilities of the terrorist organisation. Smallpox, Ebola, and Marburg virus might be chosen because they have a reputation for causing a more horrifying illness. Also, the agents, that are highly contagious or that can be engineered for widespread dissemination via small-particle aerosols, make good candidates for consideration.

Following agents are likely to be used by the terrorists based on the ability and the extent of damage that can be caused.

Anthrax

Anthrax is caused by bacteria named Bacillus Anthracis. It is one of the deadliest agents to be used as a biological weapon. It has been used with food, water, spray, powders. It is completely tasteless and odourless.

Botulinum Toxin

It is caused by naturally found bacteria named Clostridium Botulinum. It can be used for contaminating food and water. It was known to have been used by Japan on Prisoners of War (POW) during the occupation of Manchuria.

Francisella Tularensis

As per a former Soviet Union scientist, this agent was used as a biological weapon against the Nazi Army of Germany by the Soviet Union Army in the Battle of Stalingrad of World War II.

Smallpox

Smallpox is considered a potential terrorist threat because the virus was declared eradicated in 1980 and the countries halted their mandatory smallpox vaccination campaigns, thus leaving the current population highly susceptible to the virus if it were to be released by a terrorist group. It is notable that the USA, after a terrorist threat review, purchased enough small pox vaccine to inoculate every citizen in an emergency.

Countering Bioterrorism

There is no way to know in advance which of the newly emergent pathogens the terrorists might employ. A viable strategy in this situation would be to link bioterrorism preparedness efforts with the ongoing infectious disease surveillance activities. This would shrink the space available to the terrorists.

The best way to fight bioterrorism is to be prepared to face a biological weapons attack. In this manner, the terrorists are denied achieving their goal of causing fear and panic; and more importantly the lives of many citizens can be saved.

The nations follow various strategies to minimise the chances of a bioterrorist attack and at the same time undertake efforts to enhance preparedness to meet the challenges should such a contingency arise. These multipronged measures call for a coordinated approach between different national agencies.

Intelligence Sharing

The aim is to preempt a terrorist biological attack by gaining information about the threat in making. For this purpose, the global intelligence agencies should operate together and share credible intelligence. Such information can be gleaned by tracking efforts to acquire technology, purchase equipment and make unwarranted contacts with scientists.

It has been claimed that the USA Department of State issued a warning about the work at Wuhan Institute of Virology on coronaviruses in bats and the potential for a leak therefrom as well as the possible transmission to humans. Regrettably, the US intelligence agencies failed to keep a tab on the developments at this institute. Surely with certain amount of advance knowledge, the spread of Covid-19 pandemic could have been halted in its treads at an early stage.

Partnering International Security

Renewed efforts are required to strengthen Biological and Toxin Weapons Convention, 1972 (BTWC). In absence of an exact authentication methodology to ensure compliance by the member countries, there is every chance that few countries may be carrying out research and development in their laboratories in secret. Strict verification and inspection procedures need to be put in place to prevent bioweapons programs.

There is no doubt that the individual terrorists and groups such as the Islamic State do not feel bound by international norms. And the easy accessibility and the novel features of these weapons have a pull for such elements. These state and non -state actors do not feel themselves bound by international obligations and therefore it is difficult to bind them under a regime. Yet, a collective message by international community to penalise violators may put some curbs on the proliferation of bioterrorism.

Non-proliferation and Export Control

As part of counter terrorism strategy, there is a need to enforce non-proliferation and export control on biological materials. Strict measures should be undertaken to deny terrorists access to bioweapons, their means of delivery and technologies related to their manufacture.

An international effort in this direction is being spear headed by the Australia Group, an informal group of 43 member countries established in 1985. It is a voluntary group of countries working to counter the spread of materials, equipment and technologies through export controls.

Rapid Detection

Wide surveillance and rapid detection are important for an effective response to a bioterror strike. For this purpose, pooling of human and laboratory resources along with the availability of field deployable equipment is essential. Great strides have been made in detection process through the development of biosensors using robotics and the use of artificial intelligence.

Pathogen Analysis

Rapid detection and analysis of pathogen must go hand in hand to minimise the adverse effects of a biological agent strike. The facilities should be available for speedy evaluation of a range of biological agents. At the same time, scope for raising false alarms must be minimised.

Biodefense Measures

These measures are discussed in detail in the chapter on Bio Security. These range from developing vaccines and stockpiling of the same to training the first responders. All these efforts require quick flow of information and coordination amongst different agencies. These efforts can prove very crucial in containing the spread of the pathogen.

Military Preparedness

The military, having carried out its own threat assessment, creates a state of preparedness to meet the challenges of a possible biological attack. The front line troops are provided with individual protective gear to ensure personal safety. In the event of there being casualties due to a biological agent strike, casualty evacuation and health management is activated under the supervision of medical teams. All these efforts are backed by an elaborate bio surveillance network and staff coordination in the theatre of operation. Equally important are the standard operating procedures produced with great diligence, which act as a guide for various activities and responses.

Thus, the military always has a template ready to respond to the contingencies arising out of a biological weapons strike. This knowledge and some resources at a pinch can be shared with the civil authorities in times of need. Such joint efforts can become part of quick response teams as part of the national disaster plans.

Response to Bioterrorism Attack

It is of paramount importance that early detection and response systems are in place at all times as part of the preparedness efforts. Any delay or stagnation in this process will lead to a large number of people getting affected by the pathogen attack. While the patients will overwhelm the available medical facilities, the spread of the disease will in the meanwhile remain uncontrollable.

Seeking Military Assistance

As per the current procedures, civil contingencies are to be handled primarily by the civilian agencies, with the help of paramilitary forces if required. But, a bioterrorism is a special contingency and it is recommended that assistance of specialised military teams should be sought early. This will greatly help in containing the spread of disease, as well as enable scaling up of control measures.

Usually, the military forces have a certain degree of preparedness in place to meet the challenges of biological attack on the front line. They create a surveillance network based on biosensors; establish pathogen analysis facilities in field hospitals and communication system to notify troops in vicinity about a bio-attack so that preventive measures can be immediately initiated. There is a proper system for treating and evacuation of sick persons. To maintain uniformity of action across board, detailed SOPs are issued. This template with due modifications can be adopted by the civil authorities. In any case, a close liaison between military and civil authorities is essential to tackle all challenges posed by a pandemic or a bioterrorist attack.

Public Health Facilities

A comprehensive public health response to a biological terrorist event involves epidemiologic investigation, medical treatment and prophylaxis for affected persons, and the initiation of disease prevention or environmental decontamination measures. There is a need to develop protocols towards diagnosis and management of such suspected attacks.

First responders will mostly be the Primary Healthcare Centres. Their resources have to be strengthened to meet the challenge. While there are numerous biological agents, the preparedness efforts can be focused on agents that might have the greatest impact on health and security. They would be the first ones to take note of any unusual adverse health happening and these first reports when collated at higher level will provide the complete picture. Therefore, close coordination between Primary Healthcare Centres, District Hospitals and State Health authorities can go a long way in mitigating the impact of a biological attack.

Integrated Efforts

An effective response to a biological event can be ensured through the combined efforts of different agencies like: civil administration, healthcare agency, police force, military support system, scientific bodies, local population and political leadership. Their roles have to be clearly defined and regular practices must be held to update everyone's knowledge on the subject.

Communications

Generally, this becomes a weak area when multiple agencies are involved. The lack of cross communication dilutes the efforts towards controlling the spread of the disease. Also, reliable communication links have to be made available between front line health providers and the public health officials. In this regard, help can be taken from military communication agency as it has extensive national communication network. Speed of communication plays an important role in handling all kinds of health crisis.

Resource Deployment

Certain resources can be pre-positioned as part of preparatory efforts. However, in the eventuality of a terrorist biological attack, some emergency redeployment may have to be done. Supply of critical medicines can run short or equipment like ventilators may have to be relocated and Oxygen may have to be transported from different Geographical locations. In times of crisis, optimal deployment of resources becomes a critical factor.

Recent Concerns

There is legitimate concern that bioterrorism is likely to get encouragement from the demonstrative effect of Covid-19 pandemic. Global economy was shaken to the core, lives of the people disrupted, large number of deaths and still bigger was the number of people requiring medical care, high transmissibility of the disease – these are the very set of conditions that the terrorists would want to create. Having caught their eye, it can be expected that the terrorist organisations must be trying to seek this capability.

Another aspect of Covid-19 pandemic that holds great appeal to the terrorists is that the efforts to establish the origin of the virus have not been successful. There is confusion around the possibility of its leak from a research laboratory or a natural disease outbreak.

The other area of concern is the dual use dilemma of advances in the field of biotechnology. Technologies like CRISPR are promising customised pathogens at low costs. The technology and equipment can be easily acquired disguised as efforts to produce new biotechnology products for commercial use. To thwart such efforts on part of the terrorists, all aspects of biosecurity have to be strengthened with greater international co-operation.

To Sum Up

Traditional engagements are giving way to asymmetric warfare and complex operations other than war. At the same time, terrorist activities continue to pose a threat to peace and security in different parts of the world. In both cases, the reliance in the past was primarily on conventional weapons. However, this is set to change. The employment of biological weapons offers many advantages for conducting asymmetric operations and bioterrorist attacks. These are likely to become an attractive alternative compared to the use of conventional weapons.

Biological weapons are well suited for covert operations since the pathogens take time to incubate and spread the disease. Also, small quantities of the biological agent can be infiltrated into the target area. The access to the technology for producing biological weapons can be made under dual – use cover. Recent advances in molecular sciences have the ability to enhance many harmful characteristics of these agents.

With increased likelihood of biological weapons being used in asymmetric warfare and by the terrorists, the states need to develop a cohesive response strategy. The latter should aim to prevent bioterrorists from getting access to relevant technologies and to respond robustly should there be a biological weapon strike. Public health authorities and other national agencies need to work in a synergised manner to contain and manage the effects of the attack. Military forces possess sufficient expertise in this field and should be co-opted in the early stages to give a head start to the efforts.

Bio Security – *The Challenges and Responses*

The biological events have the catastrophic potential to cause loss of life, sustained damage to the economy, societal upheaval and adverse impact on national security. Such biological threats can be manmade biological weapons or naturally occurring diseases. Biosecurity is the strategy and systems put in place to safeguard and protect a nation and its citizens against the catastrophic effects of a biological event.

Biosecurity refers to measures that are taken to stop the spread or introduction of harmful organisms to human, animal and plant life. The measures taken are a combination of processes and systems that have been put in place by bioscience laboratories and Government agencies.

Since, the concept of biosecurity emanated from agriculture, its scope and implementation was quite limited. Later, as the concept embraced human health, the scope became much wider and more comprehensively stated. Alongside, many gaps were noticed in the understanding of requirements and execution of the policies. There are many strands to biosecurity – biodefence preparedness, intelligence, trust and transparency, global cooperation and compliance, safety of research laboratories, genetic research and innovation, threat assessment etc.

Biosecurity as a defense against biological warfare, bioterrorism, and pandemics has been under-emphasised in national and international security agenda. However, Covid-19 pandemic has demonstrated to the world its destructive potential and has painted a vivid picture of what a biological war would look like. In fact, the pandemic and the biological weapons strike require similar resources and effort to combat the situation. It could be said that:

"What is good for military defence during biological warfare, is good for biosecurity during a pandemic. Vice- a —versa is equally true."

Agriculture and Livestock

Both agriculture and livestock resources are integral part of national security. Agriculture forms 20 percent to 50 percent of gross national product of many countries. Nearly 15 percent to 40 percent of the workforce in these countries is employed in agriculture. Therefore, any major adverse impact on national agriculture productivity will hugely affect the national security. The economic stability of the country depends on a bountiful and safe food supply.

The potential threat to agriculture and livestock can come from a number of pathogens. To name a few: wheat rust, soya bean rust, ear rot, karnal bunt, ring rot, bacterial blight etc. for different crops. Similarly, the threats to livestock include foot and mouth disease, African swine fever, rift valley fever, sheep and goat pox, bluetongue, lumpy skin disease etc.

With food security being of prime importance, the likelihood of attack with biological agents creates a big vulnerability. Further, such attacks could be combined with biological attacks against the human population. There are biological agents in whose case it is very difficult to distinguish between natural outbreaks and deliberate use by terrorists or non-state actors.

Recently during October 2021 there has been a recall of red, yellow and white onions, which were exported from Mexico to the USA. These are reported to be the cause of 625 people falling sick with Salmonella. While this event is being treated as a case of food contamination, it could as well have been part of a deliberate bioterrorist act.

All this goes to emphasise the urgent need to put in place a proper biosecurity strategy for agriculture and livestock and the need to create suitable surveillance and control systems.

Objectives of Biosecurity Strategy

In order to adequately address the future biological threats to national security, it is essential that a national biosecurity strategy be formulated.

Once the objectives of such a strategy have been defined, the state should development systems, organisations and put in place measures for the implementation of the strategy. These are considered below:

1. ***Risk awareness and Informed Decision making.*** The system should build risk awareness at the strategic level through analyses and research efforts to characterise deliberate, accidental and natural biological risks.

2. ***Develop Capabilities to Prevent Bio incidents.*** The state should strengthen biosecurity to prevent hostile players from obtaining or using biological material, equipment and expertise. Alongside, it should prevent the outbreak and spread of naturally occurring diseases and minimise the chances of laboratory accidents.

3. ***Preparedness to Reduce the Impact of Bio incidents.*** This would require a strong science and technology base, robust public health infrastructure and various response capabilities.

4. ***Timely Decision Making.*** For ensuring rapid response at all levels, there would be need to network, to share information, take decisions and communicate the same.

5. ***Recovery Post the Incident.*** Effective and prompt measures to be taken to restore critical infrastructure, to mitigate the adverse effects and to build public confidence.

Factors Influencing Biosecurity

Biological threats have the potential to kill millions, cost billions in economic losses, and create political and economic instability, whether naturally occurring, accidental, or man made. Consequently, biosecurity issues have acquired an ever-increasing international profile. With increasing public awareness of the impact of adverse biosecurity events and interventions, political and social demands on government regulatory agencies are growing. Some of the factors that affect biosecurity are mentioned below:

➢ Globalisation, an interconnected world.

➢ New agricultural production and food processing technologies.

➤ Increased trade in food and agricultural products.

➤ Increasing travel and movement of people across borders.

➤ Advances in communications and global access to biosecurity information.

➤ Greater public attention to biodiversity, the environment and the impact of agriculture on both.

➤ Shift towards global biosecurity architecture.

➤ Scarcity of technical and operational resources.

➤ High dependence of some countries on food imports.

Biosecurity – Effective Responses and Measures

All of the above factors project an urgent need to strengthen biosecurity, reduce biological risks posed by advances in technology, create new approaches to improve infectious disease surveillance, and thus strengthen national health security capabilities.

Bio Defence Strategy

A national biodefence strategy must be put in place; it will provide a framework around which multiple agencies can function in an effective manner to face a bio contingency. The goal of the biodefence strategy is to build preparedness for reducing the effectiveness of a biological attack and thus deter the potential attacker from employing a biological weapon. A robust defence against the most threatening agents and further improvements in vaccines, detection, physical defence, diagnosis and surveillance could create sufficient uncertainty in the minds of a potential attacker about success of its biological strike.

Alongside, substantial investment must be made in stockpiling vaccines and other medicines, research and development efforts. The local public health and medical communities and military units need to work in close coordination to detect and respond to a biological attack. The state should be able to harness the biodefence potential of government bodies, private health institutions, industry and non-governmental organisations. At the diplomatic level, provisions of the Biological Weapons Convention 1972 may be invoked to build international consensus for condemnation of any biological threat developing in the neighbourhood.

Threat Assessment

Biological threats can be manmade biological weapons or naturally occurring diseases such as novel coronavirus Covid-19. The sheer diversity of biological weapons presents major problems in detecting, characterising, and responding to such threats, particularly because they may be used in covert attacks. There are about 48 organisms that could be used offensively--25 viruses, 13 bacteria and 10 toxins.

Contemporary concerns about biological threats do not simply involve possession or non-possession of biological weapons. Instead, concerns primarily involve the degree to which states have the capacity and intent to threaten or perpetrate a biological attack. Any state with a reasonably advanced pharmaceutical and medical industry has the capability of mass-producing biological weapons. This duality also leads to problems with determining which countries have biological warfare programs.

Further, with certain organisms, only a few particles would be needed to start an infection that could potentially cause an epidemic. With a few particles of Hanta virus many thousands of people could become carriers that infect thousands more people. Also, the delivery of a biological agent can be achieved through innocuous means. All these factors make it difficult to carry out a specific advance threat assessment.

At the strategic level, the risk awareness can be built through analyses and research efforts to characterise deliberate, accidental and natural biological risks. At the operational level, biological threat assessment can be aided through surveillance and detection activities. At both levels, intelligence acquisition will play a major determining role in identifying potential biological threats. Hence, it is important that the state has a well-structured mechanism to carry out a proper threat assessment and communicate the same to the decision-makers.

In absence of reliable intelligence, governments may engage in worst case planning and thus commit exaggerated amount of resources. There is a need to guard against such tendencies, and innovative strategies may be devised to dilute the likely threat.

Situational Awareness

Situational awareness involves understanding the disease and tracking its spread through the communities. Getting the correct picture is essential for decision making and initiating appropriate actions. For this purpose, emerging data has to be collected through various means of surveillance. And then this data has to be analysed to make meaningful deductions. Integrity of the data must be maintained, for this purpose training of the staff at primary health centres and other healthcare nodes is essential. Artificial intelligence and other analytical tools may be employed to improve the quality of analysis and decision making.

Public Communication

The effective implementation of interventions during a pandemic relies on public education and cooperation, supported by an appropriate communications strategy that includes active community participation to ensure public trust. The information available on the Internet and online social media play an important role in public communication. There is big chance of misinformation being dished out. Designated national and international authorities must periodically brief the public on the current status of the disease and the level of sickness. Transparency should be the order of the day.

Bio Detection

Bio detection is a general term that encompasses the strategies put in place for the detection of biological threats. Biological threats are pathogens, infectious disease, and biological weapons that can infect significant human populations. The emphasis is on developing technologies and equipment, which provide accurate and speedy detection of the pathogen and correct disease diagnosis. New technologies are being developed to integrate bio-detection platforms with smartphone devices and extend the sensing range to the hands of ordinary individuals.

An ideal bio-detection system should have broad threat coverage to cover all human health threats (aerosol, food, water, etc.). It should imbibe high reliability and probability of detection. Also, it should have low alarm rates. The detection process should be fast enough to enable responses that mitigate the impact of attack. Timely detection and response can lead to more rapidly dispensing medical countermeasures that save lives.

The current bio detection systems incorporate integrated pathogen detection and analysis systems. There are autonomous pathogen collect/detect systems with sample processing, real-time analysis and remote reporting. Special care is needed to eliminate false reporting.

Biological Laboratory Safety

The pathological agents may be collected, grown, stored or handled in clinical laboratories, diagnostic facilities, public health laboratories, research centres and production facilities. All of these facilities are at risk of biosecurity incidents.

Laboratory biosecurity involves responsibility for the protection, control and accountability of biological materials within the facilities to prevent their unauthorised access, theft, misuse, loss, or intentional release or exposure. Misuse refers to the use of biological materials for inappropriate or illegitimate purposes. Non-state actors may attempt to penetrate these facilities for acquiring small quantities of biological agents. Proper security at these installations is of utmost importance.

Another major concern pertains to the safety issues of bio containment at these laboratories. For instance, in August 2019, the U.S. government shut down its Army Medical Research Institute of Infectious Diseases in Fort Detrick due to safety concerns. No detailed information was given for the "national security" reason. In Anhui Province, two Chinese researchers exposed to SARS in 2004 spread the disease to others, killing one.

In the case of Covid-19 pandemic, grave concerns have been expressed about the likely leak of SARS CoV-2 virus from Wuhan Institute of Virology, a PSL-4 laboratory. This being the highest safety level laboratory, the suggested leak reflects laxity in implementation of strict guidelines in handling biomaterials. Normally, laboratories with safety level 3 or 4 are used for scientific work on pathogens.

Public Health Infrastructure

The major focus of the public health system is to prevent disease in a community. To best prevent disease, knowledge of existing disease rates, risk factors, and the effectiveness of preventive measures is necessary. The first step in gaining this knowledge is to develop a surveillance system that rapidly allows public health practitioners to know the health status of the community.

Generally, most infectious disease surveillance systems are passive and rely on practitioners voluntarily reporting to the public health system, and they are often not sufficiently sensitive or timely to be of great value in terms of controlling outbreaks. This problem is best managed through conducting regular training programs.

A robust public health infrastructure should play an important role in preparedness efforts and responding in emergency situations. The primary health centres and the district hospitals have to be equipped to undertake the distribution of antibiotics and to organise vaccination programs.

To meet these challenges, the organisation has to draw detailed plans and allocate resources. The manpower has to be trained to handle bio emergencies and to learn to handle the excessive demands on the system that are likely to arise. The public health agencies will need to work with technology driven devices for the purpose of surveillance, diagnosis, analyses, collection of data and the dissemination of information. The likelihood of occurrence of infectious diseases and inadvertent/deliberate bio incident is on the increase. The state must allot sufficient financial, material and human resources towards developing strong public health systems.

Medical Resources

Medical fraternity has a major role to play in all stages of biosecurity. Therefore, harnessing these medical resources can go a long way in mitigating the effects on a bio incident. This may include devising rapid diagnostic procedures, new medical treatment strategies, hospital response policies etc. as mentioned below.

> Awareness and Education – Medical professionals should be able to recognise the diseases caused by biological agents. The professional education and training curricula should be enhanced accordingly.

> Laboratory Diagnosis – Medical professionals will be called upon to confirm through diagnostic methods the possible occurrence of a biological incident. The matter would be presented to them as an unusual pattern of sickness among certain section of population.

> Treatment and Intervention – In case of confirmation of a biological attack, medical professionals will be required to provide treatment and intervention strategies for the ill and for those exposed.

> Hospital Response – The hospitals will be overwhelmed in the event of a biological incident. There will be a large number of sick and dying. Human and material resources will be overstretched. Under these circumstances, well worked outpatient care policies and contingency planning can be of great help.

> Scientific Research. This is a continuous process. The medical community must encourage clinical studies in the area of infectious diseases, particularly those having a bearing on biosecurity.

Impact of Digital Technologies

A number of countries, including India, have been using mobile phone tools and data sources for surveillance activities during Covid-19 pandemic. These include tracking infections and community spread, identifying populated areas at risk, and enforcing quarantine orders. The digital technologies are facilitating the mammoth task of vaccinating large populations.

However, the benefits that mobile phone–enhanced public health surveillance program tools provide are also accompanied by the potential for harm. There are significant risks to citizens from the collection of sensitive data, including personal health, location, and contact data. People whose personal information is being collected might worry about who will receive the data, how those recipients might use the data, how the data might be shared with other entities, and what measures will be taken to safeguard the data from theft or abuse. Necessary safeguards must be planned and incorporated in the system.

Digital technologies cannot operate in isolation and need to be integrated into existing public healthcare systems For example, South Korea and Singapore successfully introduced contact-tracing apps to support large teams of manual contact tracers.

International Efforts

It has long been realised that the steps to contain potential bio threats can become more effective if there is a common understanding and collaboration at the international level. Foremost amongst these is the adherence to the provisions of Biological Warfare Convention 1972. According to this treaty, each member state undertakes not to develop, produce, stockpile or otherwise acquire microbial or other biological agents. However, the treaty has met with partial success due to lack of verification enforcement. Also, no viable solution has been found to the dual use dilemma. Notwithstanding the lack of cooperation in the past, there is now a renewed push to strengthen this treaty in view of the world wide havoc caused by Covid-19 pandemic.

A big contributor in the global effort can be the willing participation of the nations of the world in sharing intelligence pertaining to the efforts of the terrorist organisations and non-state actors towards acquiring biological weapon capability. The openness, transparency and trust will help boost international efforts to contain the menace of biological weapons. Also, a strict export control as envisaged by the Australia Group is another positive step.

Future Directions

The rate at which the life sciences and its associated technologies are progressing and the knowledge of the processes of life at the molecular level is advancing, highly infectious and virile pathogen are likely to emerge. The next pandemic may produce a picture much more devastating than Covid -19 pandemic. Similarly, the new tailored biological agents may totally transform the concept of biological warfare. On the positive side, these very technologies like CRISPR and synthetic biology can help to develop vaccines in accelerated time frame. In such a scenario, bio security measures assume great significance.

On the other hand, much work needs to be done in the field of bio detection by developing biosensors with greater sensitivity and precision. Using artificial intelligence techniques, it should be possible to warn of an impending bio threat on an almost real time basis.

Digital technologies have played a prominent role in managing Covid-19 pandemic in the global arena. These have been used to identify cases and clusters of infections, rapidly trace contacts, monitor travel patterns during lockdown and enable public health messaging at large scale. Looking ahead, for greater efficiency and prompt response, the public health system has to harness the power of digital technologies in order to operate as a smart system.

Because of the wide spectrum of potential biological hazards, the efforts to manage the risks should be multi-disciplinary, multi-sectoral, and above all, coordinated. Such an approach will ensure optimal utilisation of resources and addressing the impending biological threats in a holistic manner.

Biological Warfare Programs of Major Powers – *An Open Secret*

During the past century, the progress made in biotechnology and allied fields has simplified the development and production of biological weapons. In addition, genetic engineering holds perhaps the most dangerous potential. Ease of production and the broad availability of biological agents and technical knowhow have led to a further spread of biological weapons and an increased desire among the developing countries to have them.

Understanding the risks that biological weapons pose today requires a closer look at how states have historically weighed their benefits and drawbacks. Since 1945, only six countries have publicly admitted developing biological weapons, although sufficient evidence exists to suspect a dozen or more. Each state has pursued these weapons for a number of different reasons.

Global biosecurity efforts are focused on the compliance with the terms of Biological and Toxins Weapons Convention, 1972 (BTWC). Since, this treaty lacks effective monitoring mechanism, there have been flagrant violations. Based on the information available in the open domain, the efforts and programs for developing biological weapons by major powers have been documented below. The experiences and perceptions of Covid-19 pandemic are expected to further boost interest of many countries in biological warfare.

Soviet Union/Russia

The most striking feature of the Soviet program has been that it remained secret for a very long time. The Russian government asserts that it does not maintain a stockpile of biological weapons or engage in any illegal development or production activities. As the legal successor of the Soviet Union, Russia inherited its status as a party to the Geneva Protocol and the BTWC in 1992.

Soviet biological weapons program developed during two distinct phases. First phase began around 1928 following the signing of Geneva Protocol, 1925. It was based on naturally occurring pathogens that caused epidemics during World War I.

The second phase commenced around 1972, with a complete shift in research and development of biological weapons. The new approach was guided by the recent advances in genetic engineering, which enabled creation of novel, highly virile and more infectious strains of bacteria and viruses. These were considered to be many times more powerful for military purposes as compared to natural pathogens. Another matter of great coincidence was that in USA, President Richard Nixon issued an executive order on November 25, 1969 terminating the US offensive biological weapons program.

Following the break up of Soviet Union, President Boris Yeltsin of Russia ordered the cessation of the offensive biological weapons program. However, the program in some form or the other continued despite these orders; it is not known whether it was deliberately permitted or happened without the knowledge of political hierarchy.

In 1971, smallpox broke out in the Kazakh city of Aralsk and killed three of the ten people that were infected. It is speculated that they were infected by the virus from a biological weapons research centre located on a small island in the Aral Sea. In the same area, on other occasions, several fishermen and a researcher died from plague and glanders, respectively.

In 1979, the Soviet secret police orchestrated a large cover-up to explain an outbreak of anthrax in Sverdlovsk, with poisoned meat from anthrax-contaminated animals sold on the black market. It was eventually revealed to have been due to an accident in a biological weapons factory, where a clogged air filter was removed but not replaced between shifts.

In 1988, Nikolai Ustinov, a Soviet bioweapons researcher, accidently injected concentrated Marburg virus into his thumb – he died less than 3 weeks later. During his autopsy, a pathologist became infected after an accidental needle stick and died in approximately 6 weeks. The virus was collected from these patients and was reportedly weaponized. It was called "Variant U," after Dr. Ustinov.

As revealed by Dr Alibek on his defection to the West, the Soviet Union established Biopreparat, a gigantic biological warfare project that, at its height in 1995, employed more than 50,000 people in various research and production centres. The size and scope of the Soviet Union's efforts were truly staggering: they produced and stockpiled tons of anthrax bacilli and smallpox virus, some for use in intercontinental ballistic missiles, and engineered multidrug-resistant bacteria, including plague. They worked on haemorrhagic fever viruses, some of the deadliest pathogens that humankind has encountered.

With the collapse of the Soviet Union, most of these programs were halted and the research centres abandoned or converted for civilian use. Nevertheless, nobody really knows what the Russians are working on today and what happened to the weapons they produced. Many security experts now fear that some stocks of biological weapons might not have been destroyed.

Russia's military doctrine considers the possibility of limited use of nuclear weapons as well as biological weapons at the tactical and operational levels. The latter is expected to produce a strong psychological effect on enemy personnel and thus suppress their will to resist. It has been observed that gradually biological warfare is gaining traction on account of advances in biotechnology. Particular in the context of hybrid warfare, the use of biological weapons offers major advantage in terms of secrecy and deniability.

Like any country with significant pharmaceutical and biotechnology sectors, Russia possesses significant dual-use life sciences infrastructure and expertise that could be applied toward an offensive biological warfare program. This dual-use dilemma is further exacerbated by the fact that the USSR covertly operated an offensive biological warfare program in contravention of the BWC 1972 treaty. Also, of concern is that the Russian military may still possess both stockpiled biological weapons and production capacities.

China

Even though assessing China's military capabilities is notoriously difficult due to the level of secrecy and opacity that its institutions maintain, a combination of historical records, assessments, and studies provide an insight into its biological warfare programs. China possesses an advanced biotechnology infrastructure giving it the capabilities necessary to develop, produce and weaponise biological agents.

China's earliest experience with biological warfare was during the Second World War when the Japanese, through their Unit 731, carried out biological agents attacks against them. These attacks included the use of fleas carrying the bubonic plague. A few decades later, in 1984, China acceded to BTWC, 1972. Publicly, China has stated that it has observed its obligations under the BTWC in "good faith" and that it does not develop, produce, stockpile, or possess biological weapons. These assertions, however, have repeatedly been contested.

In 1993, the US intelligence observed that two civilian-run biological research centres previously known to have produced and stored biological weapons were actually controlled by the Chinese military. In the same year, the US stated publicly for the first time that it is highly probable that China has not eliminated its biological warfare program,

While not denying the existence of a biological warfare program, China has called its military research activities defensive in nature. These activities are undertaken at Institute of Military Medicine, which is tasked with studying infectious diseases. However, it has been alleged that China has conducted offensive biological warfare research with fatal consequences. Dr. Ken Alibek, a Russian defector to the West, has claimed that in the late 1980s in Xinjiang province two epidemics of hemorrhagic fever were caused by an accident in a laboratory where Chinese scientists were weaponising viral diseases.

Recent emphasis of Chinese authorities on biotechnologies, even though innocuous by itself, has immense potential for military applications. China's National Gene Bank Data Base is one of the world's largest repositories of genetic information. While this information can be used toward developing more effective treatment plans against diseases and precision medicine, it can also be used to engineer precision biological weapons.

Further, China's National Intelligence Law and its Military-Civil Fusion (MCF) strategy will give its military access to all civilian research and infrastructure, theoretically turning all dual-use technologies offensive. MCF strategy aims to harness the capability of the country's civilian sectors, including science, and technology, to advance China's military, economic, and technological prowess.

In 1993, Beijing declared eight research facilities as undertaking defensive biological warfare research and development program. These included vaccine-producing facilities, such as the Wuhan Institute of Biological Products. Since then, another 12 facilities affiliated with the governmental defense establishment and 30 facilities affiliated with the People's Liberation Army are said to be involved in the research, development, production, testing, or storage of biological weapons.

Over the years, China is said to have undertaken research on causative agents of tularemia, Q fever, plague, anthrax and eastern equine encephalitis. There is a possibility that China has weaponised ricin, botulinum toxins, and the causative agents of anthrax, cholera, plague, and tularemia. A document in public domain shows the Chinese officials describing SARS coronavirus as heralding a new era of genetic weapons that can be artificially manipulated into an emerging human disease virus, then weaponised and unleashed in a way never seen before. 18 Chinese military scientists and weapons experts wrote this paper in 2015. It deserves to be mentioned that the cause of the ongoing COVID-19 pandemic is a coronavirus that first emerged in Wuhan, China, and was named SARS-CoV-2.

The COVID-19 pandemic has disrupted the world for almost two years now. And since the very beginning, people have questioned the origins of the virus that is causing the mayhem. Questions remain whether the virus evolved naturally or has been made in the laboratory. World Health Organisation has made a number of attempts to conclusively establish the origin of the virus, but has failed to get a definitive answer.

China's growing investment in lifesciences, looser ethics around gene-editing and other cutting-edge technology and integration between government and academia raise the spectre of genetically modified pathogens being weaponized.

China acceded to BWTC, 1972 only in 1984. Its progress with the compliance with terms of the convention has been rather slow mainly due to lack of verification mechanism. China is not a member of the Australia Group.

USA

The USA began limited research and development efforts into biological weapons by exploring the use of the toxin ricin. However, when the USA entered the war, as part of collective allied effort, an offensive biological warfare program was begun in 1942. The program included a research and development facility at Camp Detrick, Maryland (renamed Fort Detrick in 1956 and known today as the US Army Medical Research Institute of Infectious Diseases (USAMRIID), testing sites in Mississippi and Utah, and a production facility in Terra Haute, Indiana. Even after the war was over, the facilities for production of anthrax spores, brucellosis and botulism continued.

After a brief lull following end of World War II, the United States ramped up efforts to develop and manufacture biological weapons as the Cold War expanded. It included extensive new investments in research and production facilities, expansion of laboratory at Fort Detrick and a large production plant at Pine Bluff Arsenal. In exchange of pardon, some of the scientists from the infamous Japanese Unit 731 were incorporated into the biological warfare program.

During the Korean War (1950-1953), the Soviet Union, China, and North Korea accused the USA of using biological weapons against North Korea. The US program did expand during the Korean War and a defensive program was launched with the objective of developing countermeasures, including vaccines, antisera, and therapeutic agents, to protect troops from possible biological attacks. By the late 1960s, the US military had developed a biological arsenal that included numerous biological pathogens, toxins, and fungal plant pathogens that could be directed against crops to induce crop failure and famine.

In 1969, President Nixon unilaterally terminated the offensive biological weapons program of the USA through an executive order. It mandated the end of offensive biological weapons research and production and the destruction of the biological weapons arsenal. However, it allowed the research efforts for the purpose of developing countermeasures, including vaccines and antisera. The entire arsenal of biological weapons was destroyed between May 1971 and February 1973 under the auspices of the US Department of Agriculture, the US Department of Health, Education, and Welfare, and the Departments of Nature Resources of Arkansas, Colorado, and Maryland. At the same time, USAMRIID was established to continue research for development of medical defense for the US military against a potential attack with biological weapons.

A program of interest is Project 112 of the USA undertaken during 1962 to 1973. Highly classified program, it aimed at studying human, animal and plants reactions to offensive and defensive application of biological agents under different climatic and terrain conditions. It primarily concerned the use of aerosols to disseminate agents that could produce temporary incapacitation. Both chemical and biological weapons were considered to be part of broader strategy of gradual deterrence as an intermediary step to be able to limit the escalation short of resorting to nuclear weapons.

Terrorist attacks on World Trade Centre of September 11, 2001 were followed by another unnerving incident of anthrax attack on the USA. A number of letters containing small quantity of anthrax were dispatched to some prominent persons and institutions. This generated fear and panic and became major national concern over the potential for biological terrorism. Underscoring the importance of the matter, the USA has adopted a formal National Biodefence Strategy of 2018.

The USA did not ratify Geneva Protocol of 1925, but it ratified BWTC, 1972 thus committing itself to nonproliferation of biological weapons. Further, in 1985, the USA joined the Australia Group, which promotes export controls on biological warfare material.

Iraq

Sadddam Hussein initiated an extensive biological weapons program in the early 1980s, despite having signed BWC, 1972. Details of biological warfare program surfaced only in the wake of the Gulf War (1990-91), when investigations were carried out by the United Nations Special Commission (UNSCOM).

Between 1985 and April 1991, Iraq developed anthrax, botulinum toxin, and aflatoxin for biological warfare. It is reported that 200 bombs and 25 ballistic missiles laden with biological agents were deployed by the time Operation Desert Storm occurred. Also, Iraq is known to have used mustard gas and sarin against Iran and ethinic groups within Iraq during the Persian Gulf War. It has been later confirmed through the testimony of one of the important defectors that Iraq had been developing biological weapons for offensive use.

International team of experts have confirmed that Iraq no longer represents a biological warfare threat. These capabilities were largely destroyed in the mid-1990s and there was no effective effort to resume these following the withdrawal of UNSCOM inspection teams in 1998. There are no reasons to suspect that the new government has any desire to resume the WMD programs.

Iraq while being a signatory to BWTC, 1972, is not a member of the Australia Group.

Japan

Japan's biological weapons program was born in the 1930's in the aftermath of Geneva Protocol of 1925. It was one of the major programs undertaken at Unit 731 of Japanese Imperial Army. The focus was to develop weapons of biological warfare, including plague, anthrax, cholera and a dozen other pathogens. Unit 731 conducted research by experimenting on humans and by field testing plague bombs by dropping them on Chinese cities to see whether they could start plague outbreaks.

Japanese endeavors in biological warfare is marked by the extensive use of biological weapons during World War II, including wide spread attacks on civilians and crops. Japanese planes dropped plague-infested fleas over Chinese cities or distributed them by means of saboteurs in rice fields and along roads. Some of the epidemics they caused persisted for years and continued to kill more than 30,000 people in 1947, long after the Japanese had surrendered. After the war, the Soviets convicted some of the Japanese biological warfare researchers for war crimes, but the USA granted freedom to all researchers in exchange for information on their human experiments.

During the ultimate months of World War II, Japan planned to use plague as a biological weapon against U.S. civilians in San Diego, California, during Operation Cherry Blossoms in the dark. The plan was set to launch on 22 September 1945, but it had been not executed due to Japan's surrender on 15 August 1945.

Japan signed the Biological and Toxin Weapons Convention in 1972 and ratified it in 1982. It is also a member of the Australia Group and maintains comprehensive export control.

However, Japan was struck by a bioterrorism incident in 1995. A radical sect Aum Shinrikyo carried out sarin attack in the Tokyo subway and attempted to disperse anthrax form a tall building. This has led to instituting of various biological security measures.

North Korea

Very little information is available in open domain about North Korea's biological weapon programs. North Korea practices such information denial across almost all of its military activities. Also, biological weapon programs are easier to hide than most military programs as these can be easily disguised as public health programs.

Following the directive of Head of State in 1980, military in North Korea started working on the development of biological weapons. Some intelligence agencies have suggested that North Korea is performing applied military-biological research in a whole number of universities, medical institutes and specialized research institutes. Work is being performed in these research centers on biological agents like anthrax, cholera, bubonic plague and smallpox. Sporadic reports by the defectors point to testing of biological agents on political prisoners.

During the last decade, their scientists and researchers have been engaged in research to produce vaccines and diagnostic test kits for avian flu, Severe Acute Respiratory Syndrome and anthrax. Such research is not only valuable for defensive biological warfare but could also be used for offensive operations.

Given the geographical dispositions and constant hostile environment, Republic of Korea is always concerned about a likely biological warfare attack by North Korea. It is quite feasible for a small group of Special Forces to infiltrate across the border carrying small quantities of a biological agent. It poses a worrisome scenario for Republic of Korea.

While North Korea is a signatory to BTWC, 1972, it is not a member of Australia Group.

Canada

Canada's involvement with bioweapons began in 1940. It is known that a Queen's University laboratory in Ontario was weaponising anthrax during World War II and a simulated attack released bacteria over Winnipeg, Manitoba. Canadian scientists tested American chemical and biological weapons in Suffield, Alberta, throughout the 1960s. While Canada produced no chemical agents during the World War I, laboratories went to work in the Second World War. The Suffield Experimental Station in Alberta was funded equally by the British and Canadian armies from 1941 to 1946 and was involved in making and testing both chemical and biological weapons.

Canada ratified the Biological Weapons Convention in 1972. Since 1990, the Biological and Chemical Defence Review Committee has been supervising the disposal of chemical and biological weapons tested on Canadian soil. It is believed that Canada does not possess any weapons of mass destruction. However, it maintains the Canadian Safety and Security Program to research and develop defenses against biological weapons. Canada is a member of the Australia Group.

An event of concern happened in July, 2019, when a group of Chinese virologists were forcibly dispatched from a Canadian laboratory. It appears to be a case of unauthorized and improper transactions of Ebola and Nipah viruses. While little is known about the complicity of different individuals, there seems to be a connection to some military and scientific research facilities in China.

United Kingdom (U.K)

With the onset of World War II, Britain established a biological weapon program at Porton Down and shortly tularemia, anthrax, brucellosis, and botulism toxins had been effectively weaponized. British scientists studied the use of biological weapons, including a test using anthrax on the Scottish island of Gruinard. The biological agent left it contaminated and fenced off for nearly fifty years until an intensive four-year program to eradicate the spores was completed in 1990. They also manufactured five million linseed-oil cattle cakes with a hole bored into them for addition of anthrax spores between 1942 and mid-1943. These were to be dropped on Germany using specially designed containers each holding 400 cakes, in a project known as Operation Vegetarian. It was intended that the disease would destroy the German beef and dairy herds and possibly spread to the human population. Preparations were not complete until early 1944. Operation Vegetarian was only to be used in the event of a German anthrax attack on the United Kingdom.

British scientists experimented with ways of spreading foot-and-mouth disease, and lethal infections such as dysentery, cholera and typhoid in secret biological warfare trials. Offensive weapons development continued after the war into the 1950s with tests of plague, brucellosis, tularemia and later equine encephalomyelitis and vaccinia viruses. The program was canceled in 1956 when the British government renounced the use of biological and chemical weapons. In 1974, biological weapons were banned, and the United Kingdom ratified the Biological and Toxin Weapons Convention in March 1975.

While deciding to abandon the offensive biological warfare research and to destroy stockpiles, U. K put a new emphasis on further development of biological defensive research. U.K. is member of the Australia Group.

Germany

Substantial evidence suggests the existence of an ambitious biological warfare program in Germany during World War I. This program allegedly featured covert operations. During World War I, reports circulated of attempts by Germans to ship horses and cattle inoculated with disease-producing bacteria, such as *Bacillus anthracis* (anthrax) and *Pseudomonas pseudomallei* (glanders), to the USA and other countries. The same agents were used to infect Romanian sheep that were designated for export to Russia. Other allegations of attempts by Germany to spread cholera in Italy and plague in St. Petersburg in Russia followed. Germany denied all these allegations, including the accusation that biological bombs were dropped over British positions.

The aim of German biological weapons program was primarily to undermine the enemy's economic capacity to wage war.

There was widespread agreement that anti-human pathogens should not be developed. Consequently, the German program considered only anti-animal and anti-crop pathogens. BW attack by an Allied Power. The Nazis performed experiments on prisoners in their concentration camps. Prisoners were infected with Rickettsia prowazekii, Rickettsia mooseri, the Hepatitis A virus, and Plasmodia spp. Experiments were done primarily to aid in the development of preventive vaccines. The biological weapons programs of the inter-war period continued throughout World War II.

Germany acceded to BWC, 1972 in April 1983 and is also a member of the Australia Group. In 2018, a man was arrested in Cologne on charges of producing biological weapons at home. The police found highly toxin ricin in his apartment. The man had sympathies for the Islamic State. This incident confirms that there exists a real threat from the non-state actors about using biological weapons.

France

France possessed a biological weapons program from 1921 to 1926 and again from 1935 to 1940, and 1947 to 1956. The biological weapons program officially continued through 1972 though it did so with diminished funding and interest as investment and research efforts shifted to the nation's nuclear weapons program. During these periods, France weaponized the potato beetle and conducted research on the pathogens that cause anthrax, salmonella, cholera, and rinderpest. Its scientists also investigated botulinum toxin and ricin. It acceded to the Biological and Toxin Weapons Convention (BTWC) on 27 September 1984, and is a member of the Australia Group.

France is not suspected of having a current offensive biological weapons program. Under France's 1972 Law on the Prohibition of Biological Weapons, it is illegal to produce or stockpile these weapons.

Australia

The Australian Department of Defence formed the New Weapons and Equipment Development Committee soon after the end of WWII. Documents in the National Archives, declassified in 1998, revealed the extent to which Australia considered the development of biological weapons in the 1940s and 50s. It considered the possibilities of biological warfare in the tropics against troops and civil populations at a relatively low level of hygiene and with correspondingly high resistance to the common infectious diseases.

Specifically to the Australian situation, the most effective counter-offensive to threatened invasion by overpopulated Asiatic countries would be directed towards the destruction by biological or chemical means of tropical food crops and the dissemination of infectious disease capable of spreading in tropical but not under Australian conditions.

It also considered main strategic use of biological warfare to administer the coup de grace to a virtually defeated enemy and compel surrender in the same way that the atomic bomb served in 1945. Its use has the tremendous advantage of not destroying the enemy's industrial potential, which can then be taken over intact. Overt biological warfare might be used to enforce surrender by psychological rather than direct destructive measures. It has also been suggested that the biological warfare could be a powerful weapon to help defend a sparsely populated Australia.

Australia has advanced research programs in immunology, microbiology and genetic engineering that support an industry providing world-class vaccines for domestic use and export. It also has an extensive wine industry and produces microorganisms on an industrial scale to support other industries including agriculture, food technology and brewing. The dual-use nature of these facilities means that Australia, like any country with advanced biotechnological industries, could easily produce biological warfare agents. The Australian Centre for Disease Preparedness in Geelong, Victoria is researching the Ebola virus.

In its efforts to control spread of biological weapons, an informal group of 42 states has been established in 1985 called the Australia Group. It is a voluntary arrangement through which these countries, as well as the European Union, coordinate their national export controls to limit the supply of chemicals and biological agents-as well as related equipment, technologies, and knowledge to countries and non-state entities suspected of pursuing chemical or biological weapons capabilities. All participants are members of Biological Weapons Convention, 1972 and have stated that they view the Australia Group as a practical way to uphold the core purpose of the accord: preventing the spread of chemical and biological weapons.

Israel

Israel maintains ambiguity in its policy concerning weapons of mass destruction and accordingly, it has never made a public policy statement on biological weapons. Israel is not a signatory to BWC, 1972. It maintains its reticence and ambiguity regarding biological weapons research, development and deployment. However, Israeli biological defensive research work often appears in open publications.

The precarious security environment and strong scientific base would normally provide enough motivation for Israel to develop biological weapons. However, the military in the country consider these to be of limited value, as their employment on adversaries in close proximity could be risky due to the blow back phenomenon. Further, the short duration of the likely conflicts preclude the use of biological weapons, which have long incubation period.

It has been reported that Israeli F-16 crew have received training in loading active chemical and biological warheads onto airplanes. Though shrouded in secrecy, it is believed that Israel has developed an offensive biological warfare capability. Speculation about Israel biological warfare program mainly relates to Israel Institute for Biological Research (IIBR), which employs large number of scientists in the fields of biology, biotechnology, pharmacology and environmental sciences. It is a highly classified research centre funded by their ministry of defence.

Ostensibly, a dual- use technology facility, the publications emanating from IIBR suggest research work on plague bacterium, typhus bacterium, anthrax bacterium, botulinum toxin and ebola virus. There are no declared research laboratories of BSL-3 and BSL-4 categories. However, Israel has a strong industrial biotechnology base which can be expected to deliver on biological weapons front if the need arises.

While Israel maintains advanced R&D biodefense, and even possibly BW agent production capabilities, most analysts do not believe Israel maintains active production or stockpiles. In 2007, international media outlets reported that Israel had independently developed an anthrax vaccine during the latter half of the 1990s in response to a perceived Iraqi threat. While the fall of Saddam Hussein's regime removed the Iraq threat, Israeli policymakers remain concerned over the bioterrorism scenarios involving Islamic terrorist organizations such as al-Qaeda and Hizbullah. In 2010, the Israeli Defence Forces held a two-day bioterrorism drill and at the end of 2011 it conducted a series of bioterrorism and radiological terrorism simulations, which displayed Israeli seriousness about its bioterrorism response capabilities.

Take Away

Biological warfare is an emerging threat of 21st Century. Notwithstanding the ambit of BTWC, 1972, many of the major powers either have ongoing biological weapons program or are in a position to launch one in quick time. Terrorist threat is also real and perhaps is getting worse by the day. Dual-use nature of biotechnology and allied fields of science readily provide a cover of justification to the ambitions of the states in pursuing biological weapons programs.

Biological and Toxin Weapons Convention 1972 – *Disarmament and Global Security*

Traditional arms control and nonproliferation measures are significantly less successful at halting the spread of biological weapons than other proscribed weapons. Effective biological disarmament faces two major hurdles: the ease of acquiring the dual -use materials and technologies required to develop biological weapons, and the difficulty in verifying that these resources are not being used for hostile purposes.

The world is still struggling to devise an effective mechanism and treaty to promote biological disarmament. Partly, it has been due to lack of sense of urgency. There has not been a major incident involving release of a biological weapon as part of a planned strategy. Simply put, there has been no Hiroshima like experience to raise the level of concern regarding biological weapons. Even, sufficient financial resources are not being earmarked for these disarmament efforts. But, it is expected that the follow up studies on the devastation caused by Covid-19 pandemic are likely to get the strategic community to lend urgency to biological disarmament.

Background

The history of biological warfare goes back to the olden times, but it was the use of chemical weapons like tear gas by France and the Chlorine gas by Germany in World War I that prompted the drafting of a treaty prohibiting the use of chemical and biological weapons. It is called Geneva Protocol of 1925 and was the first attempt to control proliferation of weapons in these categories.

However, during the process of ratification of this treaty, its terms got diluted so that the signatory countries considered it as " no first use" agreement. A number of countries submitted reservations when becoming parties to the Geneva Protocol, declaring that they only regarded the non-use obligations as applying to other parties and that these obligations would cease to apply if the prohibited weapons were used against them.

During World War II and the Cold War period, there were flagrant violations of the Geneva Protocol. Major powers undertook the development of biological weapons and their testing on animals and prisoners of war. Alongside, the world grew aware of the potential dangers that lay ahead in the use of biological weapons as WMD. In a unilateral move, the Americans terminated their bioweapons program through an executive order by President Richard Nixon on November 25, 1969 and stated that their biological research henceforth will be confined to defensive measures alone.

This was followed by hectic negotiations among the member countries and after de-linking chemical weapons, the treaty referred to as " **Biological and Toxin Weapons Convention (BTWC)**" was negotiated in 1972. A disarmament treaty it effectively prohibits the development, production, acquisition, transfer and the use of biological weapons.

Biological and Toxin Weapons Convention 1972 (BTWC)

An arms control and nonproliferation treaty, BTWC aims to halt the spread of biological weapons. Some of the key articles of the treaty are summarized below.

Article I: Never under any circumstances to develop, produce, stockpile, acquire, or retain biological weapons.

Article II: To destroy or divert to peaceful purposes biological weapons and associated resources prior to joining the treaty.

Article III: Not to transfer, or in any way assist, encourage, or induce anyone else to acquire or retain biological weapons.

Article IV: To take any national measures necessary to implement the provisions of the BTWC domestically.

Article V: Undertaking to consult bilaterally and multilaterally and cooperate in solving any problems, which may arise in relation to the objective, or in the application, of the BTWC.

Article VI: Right to request the United Nations Security Council to investigate alleged breaches of the BTWC, and undertaking to cooperate in carrying out any investigation initiated by the Security Council.

Article VII: To assist States which have been exposed to danger as a result of a violation of the BTWC.

Article X: Undertaking to facilitate, and have the right to participate in, the fullest possible exchange of equipment, materials and information for peaceful purposes.

Negotiating a Verification Protocol

It has been observed that, unlike the chemical or nuclear weapons regimes, the BTWC lacks a system to verify States' compliance with the treaty and its effective implementation. Perhaps, the Cold War politics of that time prevented agreement on such a system. This lack of an enforcement mechanism has undermined the effectiveness of the BTWC, as it is unable to prevent systematic violations.

A long negotiation process to add a verification mechanism began in 1991 with the aim of evolving a legally binding verification protocol. These efforts continued through formation of large number of study groups, but the success eluded them. Finally, in March 2001, a draft protocol based on general agreement was circulated. However, the USA rejected the protocol citing the national security and commercial interests.

Considering the importance of the subject, in subsequent years, calls for restarting negotiations on a verification protocol have been repeatedly voiced. During the 2019 Meeting of Experts several member states stressed the urgency of resuming multilateral negotiations aimed at concluding a non-discriminatory, legally binding instrument dealing with the verification measures.

Government of India too, in a statement released on 26 March, 2020 on 45th anniversary of BWTC coming into force, stated:

"India takes this opportunity to call upon all States Parties to the BWC to recommit themselves to full and effective implementation of the Convention and full compliance with it, in letter and spirit. India reaffirms its unwavering commitment to continue to work together with fellow States Parties towards strengthening the Convention in all its aspects."

Non-compliance

The convention has been flagrantly violated in the past. A number of States have breached the Convention's obligations by developing or producing biological weapons. Because of the intense secrecy around biological weapons program, it is very difficult to assess whether a given program is in violation or is in pursuit of a legitimate defensive one. But, the events as they have unfolded leave little doubt that the violations have been a fact of life.

Through the testimony of scientists who defected to the West, it has been established that the Soviet Union operated the world's largest and most sophisticated biological weapons program. Close to 60,000 people were employed in the program in a hundred plus facilities. Similarly, Iraq violated its commitments as a signatory state with its biological weapons program that was uncovered by the UN Special Commission. North Korea, Cuba, Iran and China have also been accused of violations of the treaty. It is of concern that Israel is not a signatory to this treaty, which raises the fears that the country may be having a biological weapons program.

It needs to be noted that the core problem leading to non- compliance is that it is extremely difficult to confirm whether a State is complying with the treaty obligations. Further, there are no punitive measures specified. Thus, in its present form, the treaty is a toothless one.

Existing Ambiguities

The restriction on stockpiling of biological weapons has some built in ambiguities. As, it leaves room for stockpiling small quantities of pathogenic agents for scientific research and for defensive purposes. This was deliberately created option for the good of mankind, since the research and development in life sciences is required for vaccines and other chronic diseases.

But, what happens when such trust is betrayed. The small stored quantities of agents can be easily multiplied into large stockpiles for use in biological weapons. Further, as has been shown by the spread of SARS CoV-2 virus during Covid-19 pandemic, even a small quantity of the agent can cause a pandemic.

Further, no criteria have been laid down to differentiate offensive from defensive research, development, production and stockpiling capabilities. It simply becomes a subjective assessment, which is not acceptable. Thus, while BTWC represents significant international agreements on the means of biological warfare, its terms have been a source of contention and different interpretations.

Implications of Advances in Biotechnology

The revolution in biotechnology has transformed conventional biological warfare. Genetic engineering and synthetic biology have raised the specter of stealth weapons, binary weapons; all possessing enhanced virulence and transmissibility.

There are several reasons, which in future will make genetically engineered pathogens a weapon of choice for states and non-state actors. These reasons include: relatively cheap WMDs, easy accessibility due to dual-use, easy delivery and dispersal and the secrecy about the origin. Therefore, use of biological weapons has become an attractive strategic option.

This indeed has become a source of worry today, whether advances in biotechnology could tempt states to revive their old biological weapons programs or start new ones. Such an outcome would drastically undermine the progress of the last several decades. A revitalization of state biological weapons programs has the potential to trigger new conflicts or rekindle old arms races. This can disturb the world peace and destabilize the international order.

For individual actors who are motivated to spread their radical ideologies and would execute whatever is necessary to achieve their goals, the use of these advanced biological weapons could effectively deliver their message. The element of secrecy about the source of origin and the time delay by way of the incubation period add to their value for clandestine activities.

Faced with extremes of promise and peril, policymakers must proceed with a sense of perspective. Fear mongering or overregulation could undercut the almost unimaginable benefits of the biotechnology revolution. But failing to anticipate and manage the significant risks, including the resurgence of state biological weapons programs, would be equally problematic. Herein lies the challenge for reshaping the BTWC so that world can be made safer, without sacrificing the benefits of advances in science and technology.

Concerns about BTWC

As in the case of Geneva Protocol, 1925, the BTWC does not provide firm guidelines for inspections and control of disarmament and adherence to the protocol. In addition, there are no guidelines on enforcement and how to deal with violations. Furthermore, there are different interpretations about the definition of "defensive research" and the quantities of pathogens necessary for this purpose. What really matters is the intent of actions. And there is no straightforward method of determining the intent. Even, USA has been targeted for hiding offensive weapons research under the guise of defensive potential.

The convention stipulates that states shall cooperate bilaterally or multilaterally to solve compliance issues. However, there is no implementation body of the BTWC, allowing for blatant violations as seen in the past. There is a review conference every five years to review the convention's implementation, and establish confidence-building measures.

The alleged violations of the BTWC are to be reported to the UN Security Council, which may in turn initiate inspections of accused parties, as well as modalities of correction. The right of permanent members of the Security Council to veto proposed inspections, however, undermines this provision.

Concern about Those Outside the Ambit of BTWC

Non-state actors have undertaken many of the recent acts of use of biological agents. These include: the release of nerve gas into Tokyo subway system in 1995 by Aum Shinrikyo, anthrax letters distribution in the USA, salmonella infection in the salad at Rajneesh Ashram in Oregon and some of the covert assassinations in U.K and other countries. All these perpetrators fall outside the BTWC and therefore avoid even minimal oversight.

In the past, the strategists drew comfort in the thought that the technology, resources requirement and the uncertainties associated with biological weapons would render their acquisition an unviable option for the non-state actors. But, the revolution in Biotechnology has changed it all. The threat of bioterrorism is real and the security experts need to step up their efforts to counter the same.

Dilemma of Dual Use

The dual-use nature of biotechnology means that materials, equipment, skills, and facilities designed for peaceful endeavors can also be exploited for hostile purposes. These resources are widely available in open market and are highly sought by countries interested in economic development.

When it comes to verification, the core problem is that the capabilities for conducting research, development, production and testing of biological weapons are virtually identical to those employed by defensive programs and in legitimate civilian enterprises. Under these circumstances, reliance has to be placed on some ground indicators. Having large dedicated production plants, stockpiles of bulk agents or filled munitions are some of the indicators that can provide intelligence agencies and inspectors some clues to a state failing to meet its obligations under BTWC.

To meet the dual use challenge, a balance has to be struck between transparency and commercial confidentiality.

Periodic Review and Amendment

Every five years, the BTWC states parties gather at a Review Conference to discuss the convention's operation and implementation. The most recent Review Conference, in November 2016, was a disappointment for the majority of the states parties: There was minimal agreement on the final document, meaning there is no substantive program of work for the next five years. Some of the major issues include advances in science and technology, disease outbreak preparedness and response, and national BTWC implementation. Previously held mid-year experts' meetings have also been dropped.

The BTWC is an enduring disarmament treaty, the first multilateral treaty banning an entire category of weapons of mass destruction. It entered into force in 1975 and has 178 states parties. Eighteen states have not joined the treaty, which keeps it from being universal, and many states parties have not passed the necessary legislation to implement the treaty's provisions domestically. Nevertheless, the agreement remains a significant barrier to the development and use of biological weapons.

The treaty is now under pressure to move forward and take into account contemporary advances in genetics and molecular sciences. It needs continued strong leadership to bring it back from a disappointing 2016 Review Conference meeting, funding to ensure it remains a viable disarmament mechanism, and vision on how it can be integrated into a larger and increasingly integrated global security architecture.

Australia Group

The Australia Group is a multilateral export control regime and an informal group of countries established in 1985. It helps member countries to identify those exports, which need to be controlled so as not to contribute to the spread of chemical and biological weapons. It has membership of 42 countries and India became a member in 2018. All participants are members of BTWC.

The Australia Group establishes "control lists," and its members are expected to deny export license requests for items on the lists when there is a concern that the items might be used in biological weapons program. The members meet each year to coordinate export policies, discuss possible revisions in control lists and share intelligence concerning proliferation.

Though focused on the states, the group since 2002 has started addressing the flow of biological warfare capabilities to non-state actors. Rather than usurping the functioning of BTWC, Australia Group is considered to be another layer of control. It adds strength to global security architecture to control proliferation of biological weapons.

BTWC and Global Security Architecture

The global diffusion of dual-use technology coupled with strong incentive for revisionist states and extremist terrorist groups to harness this technology for hostile purposes, poses a severe challenge to international peace and stability in the twenty-first century. Biological threats know no boundaries. There is a constant need to strengthen national and international capabilities to rapidly identify, assess and respond to biological attacks.

In the past, international security concerns towards the biological warfare have been limited and the funding levels have dwindled. This situation needs to change, as the advances in biotechnology are fast transforming the nature and capabilities of biological weapons. In due course, these new weapons would raise fresh security concerns, particularly in the field of bioterrorism.

Despite the slow progress within the BTWC itself, there are other positive trends. Different international agencies are working to build inter-connects between biological weapons, biosecurity, infectious disease management, non- proliferation, science and technology. When such global initiatives interconnect, it reinforces all the initiatives. There is diffusion of ideas and overlap of thoughts, which provide great synergy to international efforts.

These are positive signs not only for the role the BTWC plays in prohibiting the development and use of biological weapons but also the future importance of the BTWC in the larger global security architecture.

Future Needs

Covid-19 pandemic has added to the urgency of making BTWC fully effective. Time to act is right here and now – the world needs to act in a similar way as it did during the cold war for the nuclear treaties. BTWC needs must be brought to conclusion with the same degree of alacrity.

More robust global governance of biosafety and biosecurity is needed. Such a governance should include these three key areas: a more effective ban on offensive biological warfare programs, greater preparation to tackle the menace of bioterrorism and more transparent and routine surveillance of biological research laboratories.

The supporting multilayered actions, like export controls on biological materials, through Australia Group should be encouraged. Sharing of intelligence, about likely bioterrorism activities, at the international level strengthen preventive efforts. Also, without credible intelligence, it is difficult to bring defaulting states into compliance of BTWC.

The challenge calls for creating a strong leadership with a vision to promote BTWC as part of larger interconnected global security architecture.

Covid-19 Pandemic – *The Virus Parade*

Ongoing Covid -19 Pandemic has brought home the fact that a virus can cause huge disruptions and damage to life on a global scale. The novel coronavirus was renamed SARS-CoV-2 indicating its similarity with the SARS 2003 outbreak, and the disease was named COVID -19. The speed and spread of the infection surpassed the capabilities of public health systems, even in highly developed societies. Heavy disruptions have led to severe strain on global supply chains, thus exposing the fragility of world economy.

This global health crisis demonstrates how a widespread disease can endanger not only the physical wellness of the citizens but also socioeconomic structures.

Points to Ponder

Indeed Pandemic – 19 has been an earth-shaking event, like the two World Wars. Millions of people have died; many more have fallen sick, with families left distraught and the society shaken to its core. Huge disruptions have been caused in the industrial output and the economies of the countries have nose-dived. It is natural therefore to seek answers to following questions: -

- ➢ How and why did it happen?

- ➢ Is it a natural calamity or man made?

- ➢ How did a small germ "virus" manage to put up such a deadly show?

- ➢ Will the world always remain vulnerable to such threats?

- ➢ How much did the global community collaborate to fight the menace of the pandemic?

- ➢ Lessons learnt to act as guide for future.

- ➢ Impact on national security.

Pandemic Timelines – Global and Indian

Not only was the breakout of the disease a surprise, the authorities were confounded by the speed of spread. In no time, the public health resources even in the developed countries came under severe strain. It is worth looking at various timelines, both global and Indian, in order to appreciate the situation.

- ➢ 31st December 2019: The WHO China Country Office was informed of cases of pneumonia with unknown cause. It was detected in Wuhan City, Hubei Province of China.

- ➢ 7th January 2020: The Chinese authorities identified & isolated a new type of Coronavirus.

- ➢ 12th January 2020: China shares the genetic sequence of novel coronavirus with other countries.

- ➢ 15th January 2020: Japan reported an imported case of Covid-19 from Wuhan, China.

- ➢ 30th January 2020: India reported first case of Covid-19 in Kerala. Individual had travel history to Wuhan, China.

- ➢ 10th March 2020: India reported first Covid-19 death in Karnataka.

- ➢ 11th March 2020: WHO declared Covid-19 a global pandemic.

- ➢ 17th March 2020: All countries of Europe had confirmed at least one Covid-19 patient.

- ➢ 31st May 2020: COVID-19 has spread to more than 200 countries, with nearly 6 million confirmed cases and 3,67,255 deaths.

Socio-Economic Impact

The COVID-19 pandemic has impacted almost every country in the world. In addition to causing alarming and tragic death tolls, the virus has shown the widespread social and economic havoc that a pandemic can yield.

The economic toll of Covid-19pandemin has been massive. The global economy has faced a depression, which is the deepest since the end of World War II. As per a report released by the IMF, world economy shrank by 4.4% in 2020. But, even this figure understates the cost, because it measures the world economy's fall from where it was before the pandemic and not from where it would have been in the normal course.

The total cost is estimated at more than $16 trillion. While virtually every posted a negative growth in 2020, the downturn was more pronounced in the poorest parts of the world. The only major economy to grow was China in 2020 with likely growth of 2.3%. Some experts have warned that it could be years before levels of employment return to those seen before the pandemic.

The travel and hospitality industries were the worst hit. Tight travel restrictions were imposed which are now being gradually eased. In the hospitality sector, millions of jobs have been lost and many companies have gone bankrupt. However, with the waning of the pandemic, rebound in global economy is becoming visible. But, the outbreak of the virus variants could prolong the pandemic and dampen the prospects of economy recovering.

Beyond the heavy disruption and economic downturn, there has been incalculable loss in terms of human lives lost. As on 26 November 2021, worldwide total number of deaths is 5,203,100 and sick are 260,511,421. Many more people have been pushed into poverty, lives upended, careers derailed and families torn apart. Some estimates indicate that 95 million people may have entered into extreme poverty in 2020 compared to pre-pandemic.

Global Response

On the public health front, the World Health Organisation (WHO) led the global response to the pandemic. There are mixed reactions to the performance of the organization.

In the first instance, the WHO was perhaps too cautious in declaring the risk of Covid -19. Had it been bolder, and had nations heeded its guidance, the pandemic might have been curtailed and the level of devastation limited.

Doubts have arisen about the transparency in the functioning of the WHO. Particularly, when it came to figuring out the origin of SARS CoV-2 virus, the WHO did not forcefully seek answers from China. It failed to get details of early patients in Wuhan and could not arrange for the investigating team to get access to Wuhan Institute of Virology.

There have been vast disparities in vaccinating the population; African countries are lagging far behind with only 2 to 5 percent of the population vaccinated. The WHO needs to prevail upon the developed countries to do more for the under privileged.

Looking ahead, the WHO needs to create an international sense of responsibility while undertaking advanced research in life sciences. Some kind of global guidance framework for regulating dual-use technology applications has to be worked out.

There is much to learn from the experience of fighting Covid-19 pandemic. Lessons thus drawn out must be followed up with action so that the world is better prepared to fight the next pandemic as and when it strikes.

It is a long held belief that the WHO faces severe limitations in performing its role. It has no legal power to enforce its recommendations or to demand information from a member country. Since, it is chronically underfunded and is reliant on donations from its member countries. This in turn throttles the capacity of the WHO to function in an independent manner without extraneous influence.

Treatment Protocol

A previously unknown respiratory illness, Covid-19 is caused by SARS CoV-2 coronavirus. It was declared a pandemic on 11 March 2020, nearly three months after the first case was detected in China. The rapid spread of the disease with large number of people becoming sick raised global alarm. Scientists and medical fraternity worked hard to devise a management strategy and treatment protocol for the disease.

In the beginning, treatment protocol for serious cases comprised plasma therapy and many other medicines like hydrochloroquinine. But, there were massive gaps in knowledge about the disease. One such gap related to the manner in which the virus would spread and how best to protect against it. Initially, it was thought that virus spreads as droplets: and hence surface contact was thought to be the route. This later got revised to spread of the virus occurring via the aerosols. Accordingly, wearing a mask and social distancing were considered good preventive measures.

Similarly, initially ventilators were recommended in large numbers. However, these could not raise the survivability rate. Instead, later it was the delivery of oxygen to the patient that became the predominant effort. With the passage of time, the experts and the authorities recommended different treatment protocols and patient management strategies. Thus, as the understanding of this vial infectious disease grew, system improved itself. This is a natural phenomenon during a period of uncertainty.

There is no doubt that the frontline health workers; the hospital staff and health care authorities did a remarkable job in attending to the sick. There was a great deal of global coordination in sharing of information. Of course, there is always scope for improvent and the lessons for future must have been noted.

Vaccination – the Unequal Worlds

As discussed in Chapter, it was an historic achievement to develop vaccines for immunization against SARS CoV-2 in record time of one year. Operation Warp Speed was able to draw the best out of public and private sector undertakings. The follow up manufacture of vaccines also picked up through ramping up of capacities.

However, the restricted availability of vaccines in the third world has left a bitter taste. As against 60 to 70 percent population vaccinated in developed world only about 4 to 5 percent population has been vaccinated in African countries at a given point in time. Not only that such a situation is immoral and unacceptable, it has left the world relatively unsafe.

International community is seized of this unsavory situation and is struggling to devise means to resolve the problem. It is expected that in due course the immunization program will be implemented globally. However, a mechanism has yet to be worked out to forestall such occurrences in future.

SARS CoV-2 Virus – Its Origin?

There are reports that the US Department of State issued a warning, in 2018, about the Wuhan Virology Institute's work on the coronaviruses in bats, with its potential human transmission presenting the risk of a new pandemic. It is a different matter that there was no follow up and everyone was taken by surprise when the pandemic struck.

Since the early weeks of the pandemic, there has been a talk that the coronavirus might have escaped from a laboratory in the Chinese city of Wuhan. This proposition has been taken seriously and the President of the USA ordered a fresh intelligence assessment about the origin of SARS CoV-2 virus whether it emerged from human contact with an infected animal or from a laboratory. All these investigations under the WHO or the one ordered by the USA have failed to come up with any conclusive answers. China has not allowed unfettered access to Wuhan laboratory as well as to the first few patients who contracted the disease.

There are essentially two possibilities: one possibility is the zoonotic transfer of virus across the species that happens when the wild animals are in close contact with each other and humans. Second possibility is the leak, accidental or otherwise, from a laboratory engaged in life sciences research on coronaviruses. First cause is referred to as the natural and second as man made.

The circumstances of the outbreak of the disease point towards Wuhan city, China as the start point A leak from the laboratory is only a hypothesis, based entirely on circumstantial evidence, but a plausible one. Wuhan's Huanan seafood market where Covid-19 was initially detected is ideal for zoonotic transfer of a virus. It holds live wild animals in close proximity to each other with possibilities for a human contact.

The Wuhan Institute of Virology, which is only 12 Km from the seafood market, houses a large collection of coronaviruses. It is a PS4 safety level laboratory. Because of Chinese reluctance to allow access or to share the details about the nature of research being undertaken, it has become difficult to get answers to pertinent queries. At the same time, it is worth noting that laboratory leaks have occurred in the past at many places in different countries.

Finding out the truth is not about apportioning the blame. It is of utmost importance to understand what and how did it happen. Knowing the origin and manner of transfer will help prevent similar outbreaks of disease in future. If zoonotic spillover was the cause, knowing the mechanisms could determine where changes are needed in animal handling and interaction with humans, and help in designing a global early warning system of future risks. If the virus came from a laboratory, lessons can be drawn on the transparency and safety of bioresearch.

The viruses and related diseases are not new but the spillover to humans appears to be occurring with greater frequency. These viruses are unfamiliar to human immune systems and there in lies the problem. Hence, the search for the answers relating to the origin of SARS CoV-2 virus must go on in the interest of health security.

The Virus Variants

All viruses, including SARS-CoV-2, the virus that causes COVID-19, change over time. Most changes have little to no impact on the virus' properties. However, some changes may affect the virus's properties, such as how easily it spreads, the associated disease severity, or the performance of vaccines, therapeutic medicines, diagnostic tools, or other public health and social measures.

The variants of viruses occur when there is a change — or mutation — to the virus's genes. It is the nature of RNA viruses such as the coronavirus to evolve and change gradually. Therefore, the mutations in viruses — including the coronavirus causing the COVID-19 pandemic — are neither new nor unexpected.

Since the beginning of the COVID-19 pandemic, the SARS-CoV-2 coronavirus that causes COVID-19 has mutated (changed), resulting in different variants of the virus. Few of them are called Alpha, Beta, Gamma and Delta variants. The WHO considers the delta coronavirus a "variant of concern" because it appears to be more easily transmitted from one person to another. As of November 2021, Delta variant is regarded as the most contagious form of the SARS-CoV-2 coronavirus so far.

From military point of view, variant or the mutations of a virus with desired properties are of interest to be used as biological weapons. In the instant example, these are a product of natural evolution of the virus, whereas same result can be achieved through genetic engineering and synthetic biology.

In some instances, a new virus can be completely harmless, while in others it can be devastating. When further propagated by global supply chains, what previously might have been isolated pockets of disease turn into global concerns—and in the case of the coronavirus, a global pandemic.

SARS CoV-2 Virus – A Biological Weapon?

The devastating spread of the deadly coronavirus across the globe has triggered a conspiracy theory on social media: what if the virus was really a biological weapon? And more specifically, was it an experimental biological weapon that accidentally escaped from a laboratory in China? While, the whole idea of attaching biological warfare angle to the pandemic could be part of a disinformation campaign, yet a reasoned analysis of the proposition is in order.

The complete genome of SARS CoV-2 virus is available in the public domain. Studies of the same by the scientists suggest that this virus in its present form is not a mishmash of known viruses. There is no evidence of its tempering through the tools of biotechnology. Therefore, it can be reasonably concluded that this particular virus is naturally evolved.

But, that does not rule out the possibility that the samples of this virus are held in Wuhan Institute of Virology. People's Liberation Army

(PLA) of China is known to promote research in biological agents of military value. And in this case, the coronavirus samples in Wuhan laboratory could be part of such a military project. Therefore, eventual weaponisation of this particular virus cannot be ruled out.

Nevertheless, the pandemic makes us reflect on biological threats and their consequences. Apart from the global devastation caused by the pandemic, the subject of " virus as a weapon of mass destruction" must be of great concern to the strategists planning for the future wars. Difficulty, in establishing the origin of the virus, adds to its value as a clandestine weapon. Let there be no doubts that the biological threats are real and they will not be long in coming.

Pandemic -19 versus Spanish Flu -1918

When a major adverse public health event like the current pandemic happens, scientists, researchers and health authorities look for analog or precedents to seek immediate guidelines for tackling the calamity. In this context, medical historians have fallen back on the Influenza Pandemic 1918-20, also known as Spanish Flu.

The influenza pandemic of 1918–20, which followed World War I, was uniquely severe, causing an estimated 50 million deaths worldwide. This pandemic happened before the advent of viral culture and very little was known about the virus until the development of polymerase chain reaction (PCR) technology. The influenza and coronavirus share basic similarities in the way they're transmitted via respiratory droplets. The lessons from efforts to mitigate the spread of flu in 1918-19 have guided some of the current pandemic's policies such as physical distancing and wearing of masks.

In the recent past, the scientists have reconstructed the genome of the extinct Spanish flu virus using reverse genetics. They have identified the genes, which were essential for optimal virulence. As regards the spread of the disease, it is believed that the virus was carried around the world by the soldiers of different countries participating in World War I. In the end, the virus receded perhaps due to the changes in the strain itself, the herd immunity and the large number of deaths.

However, the researchers are of the opinion that it is hard to chart the future spread of SARS CoV-2 virus by co-relating it to Spanish Flu virus.

From, military point of view, it is of significance to study Spanish Flu virus 1918. While there are instances of use of biological agents during World War I, the general conclusion is that the virus occurrence was a natural phenomenon and not a biological weapon. This is based on the simple premise that the molecular sciences were not at an advanced stage of study at that time.

But, a significant deduction may be drawn from the occurrence of the two pandemics (1918 and 2020) that the virus can be developed as a potent biological weapon capable of causing mass destruction. In both cases, the virus caused huge number of human deaths crippling the socio-economic life of the nations around the world.

Military Learning

The devastation caused by the ongoing pandemic holds remarkable resemblance to other threats to national security. Apart from the loss of human lives, the socio-economic life has been heavily disrupted and there has been great stress on the emotional and health state of the society. It has been nearly a warlike scenario.

In fact, pandemic can be treated as a realistic biological warfare simulation. Many useful lessons can be drawn for planning and preparedness to meet such an eventuality. There can be no doubt that the militaries of the world would have undertaken a number of studies to identify the areas of concern. There is much to learn both at the strategic as well as operational levels. For India, China is a perpetual biological warfare threat in being which must be addressed with utmost diligence.

There is a point of view that the fighting the pandemic is a civilian effort managed by the government with hardly any role for the defence forces. Hence, bioterrorism attacks, if any, in future will be handled in a manner similar to managing the pandemic. Such thought process could be misplaced because pandemic was a global phenomenon and much of the guidelines were emanating from the WHO and the US

Health Agencies. Also, the initial spread of the disease in the USA and Western countries gave lead-time for other countries to prepare themselves. But, a bioterrorist event will be an isolated one and confined to a territory. The country concerned will have to fight its own battles on the frontier as well as in the interior. It is most likely that the defence forces will be tasked to manage the bioterrorist situation initially and hand it over to civilian authorities once stabilized.

Therefore, it can be inferred that the defence forces must act as the repository of knowledge on biological warfare and extend the same to fight a pandemic. This will ensure self-sufficiency within the country and a constant state of preparedness.

A corollary to the above discussion is that there should be close coordination between the defence forces and civilian agencies so that all concerned function in an integrated manner. Regular training courses and mock exercises must be conducted to sharpen the skills of the bio- warriors.

A few areas where need for improvement have been felt during the pandemic include decision-making and unity of command, resource management, communication, and information dissemination.

Fighting Future Pandemics

With Covid-19 pandemic, world has not seen the last of the pandemics. With the shrinking of jungle space, the wild animals are spilling over to the urban areas. This in turn increases the possibility of zoonotic transfer of viruses from animals to humans. Hence, another pandemic could be around sooner than later and the preparedness efforts should continue.

During the pandemic, the WHO has appeared to function in a constrained manner with hands tied behind its back. The general impression is that the China called the shots and the actions of the WHO got distorted. This must change and the next pandemic should be an occasion for the WHO to redeem itself.

With extensive research taking place in the field of biotechnology and genetic engineering becoming commonplace, the access to manipulated virus will become easier. Non-state actors and groups with malicious intentions can cause havoc. In fact, it will be difficult to distinguish between a terrorist strike and the natural outbreak of the disease. International community needs to keep a close eye on such possibilities and take preventive measures like establishing export controls etc.

In the field of vaccination, the public and private sector in the developed world came together to develop vaccines to immunize against SARS CoV-2 virus. It is an historic achievement that couple of vaccines were developed within one year after due trials. The issues concerning disparity in the availability of vaccines, particularly for African countries should be resolved through a concerted effort by the United Nations Organisation. Equally important is to tackle the diffidence shown by a section of the society through vaccine hesitancy.

Fragility of the world economy was exposed during he pandemic. In their endeavour to flatten the curve of infected people, the governments had enforced border shutdowns, travel restrictions and quarantine in countries with developed economies, sparking fears of an impending economic recession and recession. Therefore, necessary measures need to be taken to make global supply chains more robust and the world economy more resilient.

Impact on National Security

Apart from being a serious public health issue, Covid -19 pandemic must be looked upon as an important happening with deep impact on national and international security. It took the world by surprise and in a state of unpreparedness. Need for a robust medical intelligence and surveillance system at the national level has been realized.

While, health security of the population by itself is an important component of national security, yet the pandemic jeopardized many other aspects of national security. It endangered economic stability as trade and commerce came to a virtual halt; the industries were shut down and majority of the people were surviving on their savings. This caused major unrest among the population in some countries and the political leadership was under fire. In local cases, shortage of medicines and hospital beds led to ugly incidents, becoming a law and order issue.

The pandemic has a big security message, "Beware of a bioterrorism strike, it can be equally devastating". Therefore, bio threats must be addressed with great seriousness and these cannot be downplayed simply because it has not happened before.

Summing Up

One-way to describe Covid -19 pandemic would be:

"Battlefield was everywhere and everyone was fighting to win the battle."

It was a battle fought at the individual, family, city, state, national and international levels. It was a total war, which caused tremendous loss of life, hit the economy, stopped all travel, industries were closed, schools were shut and normal life was completely disrupted. If any, humanity came out as the sole winner.

Vaccines – *The Self Defence Armor*

It is of concern that one-fifth of global mortality, especially in children under the age of five, is due to infectious diseases. Vaccines have played an effective role in combating these diseases, as shown by the success of smallpox eradication, the impressive progress towards polio eradication, the significant achievements in measles mortality reduction and many others. New safe and effective vaccines continue to be developed for a variety of infections of public health importance.

Also, the military research programs throughout history have made significant contributions to medicine and, in particular, to vaccine development. Primarily the effects of infectious diseases on military conflicts have driven these efforts. To respond to the many diseases that threaten both soldiers and the public, military forces have devoted significant time and effort toward public health methods and medical research.

Lately, Covid-19 pandemic has drawn sharp focus on vaccine development process. The urgency of developing an effective vaccine got impetus with every passing day. The number of sick and dead rose alarmingly high across the globe. The scientists responded to the challenge to accelerate the process of vaccine development. In the past, vaccines took decades to create, but for Covid-19 immunisation the first vaccine was made available within one year.

With biological threats on the increase, it is important that the advances in life sciences and molecular genetics lead to faster development of vaccines in comparable time frames to the infectious disease.

History of Vaccines

The practice of immunisation dates back hundreds of years. Buddhist monks drank snake venom to confer immunity to snake bite and variolation (smearing of a skin tear with cowpox to confer immunity to smallpox) was practiced in 17th century China. Edward Jenner is considered the founder of vaccinology in the West in 1796, after he inoculated a 13 year-old-boy with vaccinia virus (cowpox), and demonstrated immunity to smallpox. In 1798, the first smallpox vaccine was developed. Over the 18th and 19th centuries, systematic implementation of mass smallpox immunisation culminated in its global eradication in 1979.

Louis Pasteur's experiments spearheaded the development of live attenuated cholera vaccine and inactivated anthrax vaccine in humans (1897 and 1904, respectively). Plague vaccine was also invented in the late 19th Century. Between 1890 and 1950, bacterial vaccine development proliferated, including the Bacillis-Calmette-Guerin (BCG) vaccination, which is still in use today.

In 1923, Alexander Glenny perfected a method to inactivate tetanus toxin with formaldehyde. The same method was used to develop a vaccine against diphtheria in 1926. Pertussis vaccine development took considerably longer, with a whole cell vaccine first licensed for use in the US in 1948.

Viral tissue culture methods were developed from 1950-1985, and led to the advent of the Salk (inactivated) polio vaccine and the Sabin (live attenuated oral) polio vaccine. Mass polio immunisation has now eradicated the disease from many regions around the world. The attenuated strains of measles, mumps and rubella have been developed for inclusion in vaccines.

The middle of the 20th century was an active time for vaccine research and development. Methods for growing viruses in the laboratory led to rapid discoveries and innovations, including the creation of vaccines for polio. Researchers targeted other common childhood diseases such as measles, mumps, and rubella, and vaccines for these diseases have reduced the disease burden greatly.

Innovative techniques now drive vaccine research, with recombinant DNA technology and new delivery techniques leading scientists in new directions. Disease targets have expanded, and some vaccine research is beginning to focus on non-infectious conditions such as addiction and allergies.

While there is ample evidence of health gains from immunization programs, there has always been resistance to vaccines in some groups. The late 1970s and 1980s marked a period of increasing litigation and decreased profitability for vaccine manufacturers, which led to a decline in the number of companies producing vaccines. The vaccine hesitancy phenomenon is hurting the immunization program for Covid-19 pandemic as well.

The Basics of Vaccination

When disease germs enter the human body, they start to reproduce. Body's immune system recognizes these germs as foreign invaders and responds by making proteins called antibodies. The first job of these is to help destroy the germs that are making you sick. They may not act fast enough to prevent you from becoming sick, but by eliminating the attacking germs, antibodies help you to get well.

The second job of the antibodies is to protect you from future infections. They remain in your bloodstream, and if the same germs ever try to infect you again — even after many years — they will come to your defense. Now that they are experienced at fighting these particular germs, they can destroy them even before they have a chance to make you sick. This is immunity. It is why most people get diseases like measles or chickenpox only once, even though they might be exposed many times during their lifetime.

The vaccines offer a good solution to this perpetual problem. They help in developing immunity without getting sick first.

The vaccines are made from the same germs (or parts of them) that cause disease; for example, polio vaccine is made from polio virus. But the germs in vaccines are either killed or weakened so they won't make you sick.

The vaccines containing these weakened or killed germs are introduced into your body, usually by injection. Your immune system reacts to the vaccine in a similar way that it would if it were being invaded by the disease — by making antibodies. The antibodies destroy the vaccine germs just as they would the disease germs — like a training exercise. Then they stay in your body, giving you immunity. If you are ever exposed to the real disease, the antibodies are there to protect you.

Thus, a vaccine stimulates your immune system to produce antibodies, exactly like it would if you were exposed to the disease. After getting vaccinated, you develop immunity to that disease, without having to get the disease first.

Trial and Approval of Vaccines

The vaccine development is a long, complex process, often lasting 10-15 years, involving a combination of public and private institutions. There are prescribed steps for development and evaluation of a vaccine. These are aimed at assessing the efficacy and safety aspects of the vaccine. Different stages of the process are considered below.

Pre-Clinical Stage

The scientists identify natural or synthetic antigens that might help prevent or treat a disease. These antigens could include virus-like particles, weakened viruses or bacteria or weakened bacterial toxins.

Pre-clinical studies use tissue culture or cell-culture systems and animal testing to assess the safety of the candidate vaccine and its immunogenicity i.e. ability to provoke an immune response. Animal subjects may include mice and monkeys. These studies give researchers an idea of the cellular responses they might expect in humans. They may also suggest a safe starting dose for the next phase of research as well as a safe method of administering the vaccine.

The pre-clinical stages usually involve researchers in private industry. Referred to as sponsor, a private company submits an application for investigation and approval of the vaccine to the National Drug Approval Authority. The sponsor, describes the manufacturing and testing processes, summarizes the laboratory reports, and describes the proposed study. An institutional review board approves the clinical protocol and then the authority grants approval for conducting three phases of testing on human subjects.

Phase I Vaccine Trials

This first attempt to assess the candidate vaccine in humans involves a small group of adults, usually between 20-80 subjects. If the vaccine is intended for children, researchers will first test adults, and then gradually step down the age of the test subjects until they reach their target. Phase I trials may be non-blinded (also known as open-label in that the researchers and perhaps subjects know whether a vaccine or placebo is used).

The goals of Phase 1 testing are to assess the safety of the candidate vaccine and to determine the type and extent of immune response that the vaccine provokes. In a small minority of Phase 1 vaccine trials, researchers may use the challenge model, attempting to infect participants with the pathogen after the experimental group has been vaccinated. The participants in these studies are carefully monitored and conditions are carefully controlled. In some cases, an attenuated, or modified, version of the pathogen is used for the challenge.

If Phase 1 trial meets with success, the process moves to the next stage.

Phase II Vaccine Trials

A larger group of several hundred individuals participates in Phase II testing. Some of the individuals may belong to groups at risk of acquiring the disease. These trials are randomized and well controlled, and include a placebo group. The goals of Phase II testing are to study the candidate vaccine's safety, immunogenicity, proposed doses, schedule of immunizations, and method of delivery.

Phase III Vaccine Trials

Successful Phase II candidate vaccines move on to larger trials, involving thousands to tens of thousands of people. These Phase III tests are randomized and double blind and involve the experimental vaccine being tested against a placebo (the placebo may be a saline solution, a vaccine for another disease, or some other substance).

Apart from the efficacy, the goal is to assess vaccine safety in a large group of people. Certain rare side effects might not surface in the smaller groups of subjects tested in earlier phases.

Licensing and Manufacture

After a successful Phase III trial, the vaccine developer will submit a Biologics License Application to drug approval authority. The latter will then inspect the factory where the vaccine will be made and approve the labeling of the vaccine.

An adverse event data collection is being done through " Vaccine Adverse Event Reporting System" (VAERS). It is a voluntary reporting system. Anyone, such as a parent, a health care provider, or friend of the patient may report an adverse experience of the patient. The report will be investigated and results collated for necessary action.

It needs to be observed that extreme care is taken during approval to ensure efficacy and safety of the vaccine. It entails a long process spanning years and huge expenditure on part of the sponsor. The latter also bears the risk of the proposed vaccine failing approval at any stage of the trials.

An interesting question at this stage is how did the USA manage to develop a vaccine for Covid-19 in a year's time when the usual process takes almost a decade.

Operation Warp Speed

The World Health Organization (WHO) declared covid-19 a previously unknown respiratory illness caused by the coronavirus SARS-CoV-2, a pandemic on 11 March 2020, less than 3 months after cases were first detected. With millions confirmed cases of sickness and large number of deaths recorded worldwide, there were grave concerns about the global health, societal and economic effects of this virus. The need for the vaccine was urgent and immediate. Measuring up to this challenge, the USA government undertook a novel initiative for development of the vaccine in a quick time frame.

The USA government launched operation Warp Speed to encourage private and public partnerships, to facilitate and accelerate the development, manufacturing and distribution of Covid-19 therapeutics and diagnostics. It was officially announced on May 15, 2020. The name "warp speed" was inspired by terminology for faster-than-light travel used in the *Star Trek* fictional universe evoking a sense of rapid progress. Operation Warp Speed was initially funded with about $10 billion.

Based on preliminary evidence, this program promoted mass production of multiple vaccines and different types of vaccine technologies, allowing for faster distribution if clinical trials confirm one of the vaccines is safe and effective. The plan anticipated that some of these vaccines would not prove safe or effective, making the program more costly than typical vaccine development, but potentially leading to the availability of a viable vaccine several months earlier than typical timelines.

Another fascinating aspect of Operation Warp Speed was the pivotal role played by the USA military. Apart from the strategic planning, it greatly facilitated operational planning, logistics and supply chains. Also, military's wide experience in contracting came handy in working out the arrangements with the drug manufacturers in a mutually beneficial manner. An Army General had then commented, "We will have trucks rolling within 24 hours of approval of the first vaccine". This is indicative of the great forethought and co-ordination provided by the military in fighting the pandemic.

Operation Warp Speed has been a spectacular success. It showed that the state could work effectively with private firms to promote innovation and provide a powerful weapon against the virus. It consisted of early and massive funding of R&D and investment in production of various vaccine candidates, as well as coordinating the value chain and addressing all regulatory and logistical hurdles. The result: several vaccines available within a year.

Covid -19 Vaccines

A Covid-19 vaccine can prevent getting the disease or from becoming seriously ill or dying due to it. Each COVID-19 vaccine causes the immune system to create antibodies to fight the disease. Covid-19 vaccines make use of a spike like structure on the surface of the SARS CoV-2 virus called an S protein. The S protein helps the virus get inside your cells and start an infection.

Covid-19 vaccines belong to one of the following main categories: -

> **Messenger RNA (mRNA) vaccine.** This type of vaccine uses genetically engineered mRNA to give the cells instructions on how to make the S protein.

> **Vector vaccine.** In this type of vaccine, the genetic material from the SARS CoV-2 virus is placed in a modified version of a different virus (viral vector). When the viral vector gets into the cells, it delivers genetic material from the SARS CoV-2 virus that gives the cells instructions to make copies of the S protein.

> **Protein subunit vaccine.** This type of Covid-19 vaccine contains harmless S proteins. Once your immune system recognizes the S proteins, it creates antibodies and defensive white blood cells. In case of infection, the antibodies will fight the virus.

The experiences in handling Covid-19 suggest that the mRNA vaccines represent a promising alternative to conventional vaccine approaches because of their high potency, capacity for rapid development and potential for low-cost manufacture and safe administration. However, there are issues concerning the logistics of delivery. Recent research shows that such problems can be largely overcome.

Covishield – A Case Study

The pandemic drew a sharp focus on the global efforts for development and production of vaccines for preventing the spread of SARS CoV-2 virus disease. The tremendous efforts devoted by the international community in a collaborative manner can be best appreciated by looking into the timelines and processes for one of the vaccines say, Covishield.

Covishield is brand name of Oxford and Astra Zeneca Covid-19 vaccine. It has been developed by Oxford University and AstraZeneca pharmaceutical company, and is given by intramuscular injection. It is a viral vector vaccine.

Serum Institute of India (SII), Pune is the world's largest vaccine manufacturer in terms of numbers. It partnered with the Oxford University to manufacture their Covid-19 vaccine in India. The SII produces 5,000 doses of the vaccine per minute in their assembly lines. Various timelines are stated below.

> April 2020: SII announced its partnership with Oxford University to manufacture their Covid-19 vaccine.

> May 2020: A 1ml vial with the cellular material for the much-anticipated vaccine arrives at SII from Oxford, England.

> August 2020: Phase-III clinical trials of Covishield began in India.

> September 2020: AstraZeneca observed a severe adverse reaction in one of the participants in their trial program and paused clinical trials in other countries. Drugs Controller General of India (DCGI) issued a show-cause notice to SII citing the failure of the company to inform about the same. The company responded saying no such effects were observed in India and the program was allowed to resume in the same month.

> November 2020: AstraZeneca declared their vaccine candidate was observed to be 70 per cent efficient based on data from trial results. It also said efficacy increased when a different dosage regimen was followed. SII announced that the company is moving to apply for an emergency use license within two weeks.

> December 2020: A trial volunteer from Chennai in Tamil Nadu reported severe adverse reaction to Covishield. SII denied any correlation between the vaccine and the condition of the volunteer.

- ➢ December30, 2020: The vaccine was first approved for use in the UK vaccination program and the first vaccination outside of a trial was administered on 4 January 2021

- ➢ January 2021: DCGI granted an emergency use approval for Covishield vaccine in India. Doses of the vaccines were transported from Pune to multiple hubs in the country.

- ➢ January 16, 2021: The first dose of the vaccine was administered to recipients based on a priority list prepared by the government.

The milestones mentioned above are testimony to the scorching pace at which public and private undertakings worked closely to provide succor to humanity in the times of the pandemic

Miscellaneous Issues

Vaccine Hesitancy

It refers to delay in acceptance or refusal of vaccines despite availability of vaccine services. There have been cases, particularly in the developed world, where vast sections of people have been reluctant to get vaccinated against Covid-19. The concerns have been expressed that such vaccine hesitancy could adversely affect global efforts at ending the pandemic.

The reasons for Covid-19 vaccine acceptance and hesitancy remain complex. These include: individual confidence, complacency, convenience (or constraints), risk calculation, and collective responsibility.

Concerted efforts are needed to alleviate the concerns of the individuals pertaining to the vaccine. The media has an important role to play. It should report in a responsible and transparent manner on the vaccine program, providing clear and unbiased information to its audiences. Equally, the authorities should be transparent about their efforts and vaccine availability. Finally, people using the Internet and social media (including scientists and clinicians) should do so responsibly to avoid spreading falsehoods or using language that could be misinterpreted and could thereby potentially add to vaccine hesitancy.

Vaccine – Disparities

Due to limited availability of vaccines for Covid-19, there have been major racial disparities in who is getting the vaccine. As of August 2021, while 80% of the vaccine doses have gone to people in high-income and upper-middle-income countries, only about 2% of people in low-income countries have been given at least one dose.

The world as a whole must commit itself to Covid-19 vaccine equity. The inequitable distribution of vaccine has allowed the virus to continue spreading. The unvaccinated populations are at risk from especially from new coronavirus variants. Guiding principle is: -

"Nobody is safe until everybody is safe".

Going Ahead

Molecular genetics has set the scene for a bright future for vaccinology, including the development of new vaccine delivery systems (e.g. DNA vaccines, viral vectors, plant vaccines and topical formulations). Therapeutic vaccines may also soon be available for allergies, autoimmune diseases and addictions. It is heartening to note that the World Health Organisation (WHO) has accorded its approval to a vaccine for Malaria on 06 Oct 2020. This should help save many lives that are lost to Malaria in many African countries.

Another suggestion, equally applicable to military and civil, is that the future vaccines should cover multiple pathogens by taking advantage of molecular genetics. This will improve the level of biodefense against hostile actors who may be contemplating a biological attack.

Advances in life sciences should be targeted towards methodologies to develop vaccine in a comparable time frame with the detection and spread of the disease. This would help in containment action and keep rest of the population safe. Also, the process of testing the vaccines must be accelerated.

India and the Pandemic – *Need For System Upgrade*

Being a developing country, India faces a host of biological threats. Its large population coupled with poor hygiene conditions in rural areas makes it quite vulnerable to infectious diseases. These have mainly been seasonal respiratory infections and water borne diseases. The cause is usually a natural pathogen and affects limited population and for a limited period. Local health professionals know various treatment protocols. Existing public health system is reasonably organised to respond to spread of such infectious diseases.

However, when SARS CoV-2 virus arrived in India, it led to mass upheaval. Primary healthcare workers were over stretched, hospitals overwhelmed with the number of patients and the society faced an emotional turmoil. While the political leadership rose to the occasion and took control of the situation, certain organisational and functional deficiencies did show up. The country would do well to plug such gaps before the next health emergency occurs.

Pandemic Strikes

The first case of coronavirus in India was reported at the end of January in the southern state of India, Kerala. The following week, three more active infections were identified in the same state. These were all traced to persons who had a travel history. With the emergence of the virus, the Ministry of Health and Family Welfare (MoHFW) took charge and tasked Indian Council for Medical Research (ICMR) and the National Institute of Virology (NIV) for the rapid development of diagnostic and research methodologies to tackle the Covid-19 pandemic.

A glaring absence at the scene of action was National Centre for Disease Control (NCDC), India whose primary role is to undertake investigations of disease outbreaks employing epidemiological and diagnostic tools. This was quite unlike the performance of a similar organisation Centre for Disease Control and Prevention (CDC), USA, where its Director was the main spokesperson on different aspects of the pandemic.

In the following months, more cases surfaced in different parts of the country, but most of them were imported with people returning to India from European regions. The havoc being played out by the coronavirus in the USA and Europe provided clear indication of the crisis looming on the horizon. Indian government took notice and acted with promptness. The Prime Minister announced a 21 days nationwide lockdown towards end of March 2020 and exhorted the people to fight the pandemic on war footing. The Disaster Management Act 2005 was invoked on 25 March 2020 and the first lockdown was imposed. In comparison to the developed countries, India was quick to implement strict social distancing policies, which paid dividends.

Broadly, India's response to the spread of SARS CoV-2 virus can be divided into three overlapping phases:

> ➢ Phase I – Controlling trans-border movement to limit infections related to international travel.

> ➢ Phase II – It involved containing the spread of disease within the country through tracing of primary and secondary contacts.

> ➢ Phase III – An overlapping action, it involved nationwide lockdown to contain local/community transmission.

With timely action, India was able to brave the first wave of the pandemic with the best foot forward; however it faltered during the second wave due to overconfidence and laxity. The pandemic impacted the socio-economic life of the citizens and caused huge loss of human lives.

On the social front, the lockdowns and social distancing have created a new normal for the families. Work from home, on line schooling and telemedicine are the new ways of life. Migrant workers suffered a great deal and faced the severest blows of the pandemic. On the economic front, post pandemic recession and large loss jobs were feared. However, the government introduced well-timed economic stimulus packages. The economy has bounced back with a near 'V' shaped recovery.

There have been 34,555,431 infections and 467,468 coronavirus-related deaths reported in the country since the pandemic began (figures noted on 26 Nov 2021).

For a country with population of over 1.3 billion, while the loss of life and livelihood is tragic, India is being lauded for its handling of the health crisis. The credit is due in large measure to the political leadership, government agencies, healthcare professionals and above all the citizens. No doubt there were gaps and lessons have been learnt for future. There is great scope for improvement.

National Disaster Management Authority (NDMA)

National Disaster Manager Authority (NDMA) of India is the nodal agency to initiate processes to alleviate strife and suffering arising out of disasters—biological, chemical, physical or hydrological. It was created under the Disaster Management (DM) Act 2005, which vested in it overriding powers to make rules and regulations for preventing, containing, evacuating, providing relief and various other related activities in the interest of the suffering public. To fight the pandemic, the DM Act 2005 was invoked on 25 March 2020, with the announcement of the first lockdown.

Apart from the imposing of lockdowns, one did not observe a prominent role being played by the NDMA. Being a nodal body for the disasters, it was expected that the NDMA would play a pivotal role in formulating an overall plan of mitigation. Perhaps, the NDMA in its present form is better prepared to handle natural disasters like floods, tsunami, cyclonic storms etc. and lacks the competence to manage the outbreak of an infectious disease.

The problem of migrant workers was of a magnitude that called for a national approach towards extending help and facilitation. The NDMA did not recognise the extent of the disaster and failed to intervene.

Bioterrorism is a real threat to India's security. Ongoing pandemic is a fairly accurate representation of the kind of devastation that a biological attack may cause. Early containment by having a state of the art bio surveillance system and organising a coordinated effort at the local level to tackle the impact must form part of disaster planning.

Following the review of its performance during the pandemic, the NDMA will do well to review its planning and preparation to meet the contingencies arising out of a bioterrorism act or natural spread of a pathogen.

Public Health System – Structure & Performance

India has a mixed health care system consisting of public and private healthcare service providers. However, most of the private healthcare providers are concentrated in the urban areas, while 65% of Indian population lives in the rural areas. The public health system in the rural areas is structured in a three- tier manner. A sub centre at the large village level, a primary health centre for a population of 30,000 people and a community health centre for 1,20,000 people. The first referral is provided at the District hospital. These public health facilities are known to be ill equipped and lack adequately trained manpower.

In the urban areas, private health providers are the active players. They provide high standard of diagnostic and treatment services, but at an exorbitant cost. Then, there are alternative systems of medicine, which may be patronised by people in non-emergent situations.

During the pandemic times, all healthcare professionals functioned with extreme dedication. Initially, they faced tremendous difficulty as the diagnostic and the public health authorities could not spell out treatment protocols, as there was a previously unknown threat. Even, it took time to provide protective clothing to the staff members. At the same time, large number of patients overwhelmed the available medical facilities.

A critical requirement arose for Oxygen gas as part of respiratory support to affected persons. Soon, supply from local sources got exhausted. There was immediate need to transport Oxygen from far-flung industrial plants in special containers. A precarious situation existed; defence forces lent a hand to manage the logistics of transportation of Oxygen and gradually the situation stabilised.

Similar, was the case in respect of Ventilators, a life saving equipment for the Intensive Care Units. There was global shortage of the ventilators, which are quite expensive as well. Thanks to the ingenuity of Indian scientists and innovators, indigenised versions of the ventilators were made available in quick time and helped save valuable lives.

There were general shortages of medicines required for the treatment and hence their distribution was regulated. In fact, under the Prime Minister's Office, a number of adhoc groups of experts were formed who functioned round the clock and were empowered to take decisions. Members of these groups frequently disseminated information on the disease through public media. This move greatly helped in dispelling any myths and generated confidence in the system. This open system of sharing pandemic information was greatly appreciated by the public.

An important point that needs to be noted is that in the case of the pandemic, bulk of the information about SARS CoV-2 virus and the treatment protocol was flowing from the WHO and other developed countries. It was so because the disease has spread in these countries earlier than India. This may not be the route of spread of disease during the next pandemic. Similarly, in case of a biological weapon strike, India may be the only affected territory. Therefore, it is of utmost importance that the public health agencies are geared to handle any bio threat on their own in the future.

National Centre for Disease Control (NCDC) – Lost Opportunity

"Missing in Action" would be an apt term to describe the role played by NCDC during the pandemic. Here is a national institute whose mandate it is to undertake investigation of disease outbreaks all over the country employing epidemiological and diagnostic tools. Yet, in the times of the pandemic, it was not anywhere on the scene.

It is worth a while to draw a parallel with similar set up in the USA, Centre for Disease Control and Prevention (CDC). It is tasked with securing global health and America's preparedness by revitalising the public health infrastructure, stopping the spread of contagious and vector-borne diseases, and addressing bioterrorism threats. It played a prominent role in responding to Covid-19 pandemic by ensuring that state and local health partners had the resources, guidance and scientific expertise to respond. It functioned 24/7 and activated its Emergency Operations Centre.

It is clear that India's NCDC failed to perform as compared to similar organisation like CDC in another country. This happened despite NCDC being an old established institution. It has its origin in Central Malaria Bureau, established in Kasauli (Himachal Pradesh) in 1909. Later, it was expanded to cover other communicable diseases. Surveillance of communicable diseases and outbreak investigation forms an indispensable part of its activities. It functions under the Ministry of Health and Family Welfare. It has a number of laboratories on its campus and various training facilities.

There is no gain saying that the NCDC has been an under utilised resource during the pandemic. If there are deficiencies, the institute should be strengthened to perform its critical role.

Global Support - Fight Against Pandemic

India received tremendous international support for fighting the pandemic. In the early part of the pandemic, India sent assistance to the USA, which was highly appreciated. However, during the second wave of the pandemic, India was hard hit and needed additional support from international community. There was wide spread international support for India's fight against Covid-19.

The WHO has been an important partner in India's fight against the disease during the pandemic. It provided timely guidance, which was helpful in containing the spread of Covid-19 across the country.

In June 2021 the World Bank approved a $500 million program to support India's large informal workforce and create greater flexibility for states to cope with the ongoing pandemic. The total funding received from the World Bank towards strengthening India's social programs to help the poor and vulnerable households affected by the pandemic stands at $1.65 billion.

Many countries including the USA, Russia, France and the U.K. rushed critical emergency use equipment to help India combat the second wave. A compilation from Ministry of External Affairs shows that large number of Oxygen concentrators, respirators and other items of medical assistance were received from other countries.

Such strategic pooling of resources goes a long way in mitigating the adverse effects of the pandemic. In addition, it helps in developing mutual goodwill among the nations.

Vaccination – Manufacture & Immunisation

Immunisation through vaccination coupled with the herd immunity is expected to put an end to Covid-19. India with a population of 1.3 billion people has an extremely challenging task of manufacturing large quantities of the vaccine, distributing the same and eventually jabbing people in far-flung remote areas. Indian Government has promised to vaccinate the entire adult population by the end of 2021.

The main stay of India's vaccination program are: Covishield and Covaxin, which are manufactured locally. The Serum Institute of India produces Covishield (under license from AstraZeneca) and Bharat Biotech produces the locally developed Covaxin. In both cases, the production capacities have been progressively ramped up to meet the huge demand.

The Covid-19 vaccination drive of India is world's largest vaccination drive and has been unprecedented in both scale and reach. India is moving with full force to meet its stated target of vaccinating the entire adult population by December 2021. Against this, the WHO has asked all countries to meet their targets to vaccinate 40% of their population by end-2021 and 70% by mid-2022.

India's laudable efforts in implementing vaccination program are best summed up in the tweet sent out by the Prime Minister, "India scripts history. We are witnessing the triumph of Indian science, enterprise and collective spirit of 130 crore Indians. Congrats India on crossing 100 crore vaccinations. Gratitude to our doctors, nurses and all those who worked to achieve this feat. #VaccineCentury."

On the world stage, India has been lauded for providing limited quantities of vaccine to its neighbours and low-income countries despite the pressing need at home. For its large manufacturing capacities of the vaccine, India is being referred to as the ' vaccine factory of the world'.

Such self-sufficiency in vaccine research and production adds to the overall national security efforts. It provides a degree of deterrence to any bio threat that may emerge in the future.

Mass Media – A Valuable Player

Mass media includes television news and interviews, Internet, social media, radio and print media. Throughout the spread and fight against the pandemic, Indian mass media played a major role in disseminating information about Government plans and policies, people's health concerns, and the facilities available for the patients.

Staying informed is the prime requirement of every individual during any calamity, and particularly so during the pandemic when every citizen's health is a matter of concern. On the whole, Indian media played an active and positive role in the country's fight against SARS CoV-2 virus. It played a major role in educating people about the nature and symptoms of the disease, preliminary treatment at home and the need to move the patient to the hospital. It emphasised hand washing, personal hygiene, wearing of masks and social distancing norms.

The government agencies made a very effective use of mass media. It was extensively used to convey the lock downs, restrictions on group activities, local rules and general healthcare policies. Keeping the citizens informed at all stages of the pandemic made them active participant in the united fight against the pandemic. Despite the loss of loved ones, the media kept up the morale of the population through motivating stories of selfless service of rendered by thousands of citizens. The plight of migrants was portrayed through candid visual images, which stirred the conscious of many.

The medical experts regularly appearing on the television to explain the nuances of the disease in layman language promoted a high degree of confidence among the people to face a difficult situation. Regular address by the Prime Minister and others in authority assured the people that every effort is being made to mitigate the hardships being faced by the citizens and that there is a sense of urgency and concern at all levels.

However, certain amount of misinformation, myths and unproven therapies by homeopathy doctors were floated on mass media. The medical experts on television made every effort to dispel wrong notions. Scientific explanations were provided to convince the viewer to make the right choices and not fall prey to vested interests.

Transparency, presentation of facts, informed discussions and objective analysis made television a popular medium. It gained on viewership from the fact that most of the people were home bound due to lockdowns/curfew etc. For the future, in the interest of national security, India must ensure that television medium is not manipulated as part of information warfare launched by an adversary. Certain amount of self-regulation by the media houses must be insisted upon.

Non-Govermental Organisations (NGOs)

Non-governmental Organisations (NGOs) have made remarkable contribution in supporting the fight against Covid-19. They primarily supplemented the state efforts and extended the reach of government agencies.

During the second wave, the Prime Minister made a special appeal to NGOs to strengthen the healthcare system. The NGOs came forward to contribute their efforts in meeting the requirement of medical grade Oxygen, in providing protective gear and in provisioning life-saving medical and diagnostic equipment. The NGOs across India played a major role in reaching out to the marginalised sections of the society. They arranged free distribution of food and provided material help to the poor.

The NGOs enjoy great trust of certain sections of the society, who are otherwise not receptive to the instructions issued by the authorities. Under the circumstances, the NGOs proved to be an effective conduit in educating the community about the precautions and hygiene measures to be taken. They made a valuable contribution in this regard.

In the case of migrants, the mass return to their villages created major logistic problems. But the NGOs and local groups came forward to serve free food and arrange resting places enroute. These efforts saved the situation, which otherwise could have been quite tragic. The contribution and the role played by the NGOs during the pandemic have received all round praise.

Harnessing of Digital Technologies

In order to generate a comprehensive and rapid response to the pandemic, India made extensive use of digital technologies. It enabled population surveillance, case identification, contact tracing and evaluation of interventions. It leveraged billions of mobile phones, large online datasets, connected devices and other computing resources.

In a large country like India, public health authorities were in know of things at all times. Apps like AarogyaSetu, CoWin were designed to be extremely user friendly so that common man could easily manage them. They were used to capture data as well as to disseminate important public health information. The whole experience has been so invigorating that it has led to accelerated research in multiple areas of digital healthcare. The future public health management will be greatly strengthened through exploitation of technologies and the preparedness to fight infectious diseases will increase manifold.

Pain of the Migrants

There are about 100 million migrant workers in India. Most of them are daily wageworkers, who have moved out from different parts of the country to find jobs to sustain their families. They were the worst affected due to the lockdowns imposed during the pandemic.

During the lockdowns, these migrants lost their jobs and left with no money. They suffered major economic setback and some were even thrown out of the rented accommodation for non-payment of rent. Many were feeding themselves at free food stalls run by various charities. Topping it all was the uncertainties about the end of the pandemic.

With passage of time, their plight became worse and exodus of reverse migration started. They decided to return to their villages using whatever means of travel were available. The shortage of transport forced many migrants and their families to undertake the journey of hundreds of miles on foot.

The NDMA failed to anticipate the looming disaster of reverse migration. No planning was done to facilitate their return or provide them with financial support to tide over the crisis. For a few days, total chaos prevailed regarding the return journey of the migrants. Also, there was no healthcare support available to the migrants and their families.

This unprecedented crisis calls for immediate looking into the needs of the migrants. Some safeguards must be built to ensure that their basic necessities are met. Affordable housing through co-operatives could be provided. National migration policies should be reworked keeping in mind the magnitude of the problem. Some special rights should be generated for them in the migrated land.

A detailed analysis of the difficulties faced by the migrants should be carried out in order to alleviate such suffering in future.

Pandemic and the Defence Forces

Beginning on 5 May 2020, Indian and Chinese troops were engaged in skirmishes and face-offs along the Sino-Indian border including the Galwan valley in Ladakh. This coincided with the onset of Covid-19 in the country. Army, which is maintaining large deployment of troops along the border, had to initiate immediate action against the spread of SARS CoV-2 virus. Large concentration of troops in one place increases their vulnerability to an infectious disease. Adding to this was the frequent in and out movement of soldiers on leave etc. So, the Indian forces were facing multiple challenges.

For obvious reasons, the data on the impact of the pandemic on the fighting efficiency of defence forces is not in the public domain. But, the fact that the forces maintained a steady stand against the Chinese and the morale of the soldiers was very high indicates that there was negligible impact if any on the fighting efficiency of the Indian military.

This observation is aided further by the excellent healthcare protocols and the high standard of discipline prevalent in the forces.

During the surge in the second wave, the defence forces chipped in with the required resources, notwithstanding their heavy commitments on the border. The warplanes to warships to ground transport were deployed to ferry medical Oxygen to meet critical shortages. Besides, military doctors and nursing staff set up many makeshift field hospitals. The tradesmen from the Corps of EME set right many oxygen plants in various locations in the states, which received much acclaim.

Despite being engaged in a war like situation with China, the defence forces made available much material and manpower resources to fight the pandemic. It is a great statement on their dedication and service to the nation.

However, there are other aspects concerning military that require consideration. The pandemic is a fairly representative reflection of what would be the situation during a biological weapon attack. The military has trained and equipped itself to face such bio threats. There are laid down standard operating procedures (SOPs) for protection of soldiers and for actions by the medical staff. Perhaps, the authorities could have tasked the forces to look after one District in any state. Apart from using it as an opportunity for live training in biological warfare, the forces would have created a model infrastructure and procedures. The latter could then have been replicated in other places.

Another thought relates to utilising the potential of defence veterans. A disciplined and trained set of manpower, they could have been embedded into the support organisations to boost their efforts.

It may be of benefit to study the role played by the defence officers in Operation Warp Speed of the USA. Their professional acumen was gainfully employed in ensuring timely development of vaccine for SARS CoV-2 virus and its subsequent smooth roll out.

Unity of Action – States and Centre

India has pushed the bar up when it comes to the centre-state unity of action during the pandemic. Indeed the national crises are the test points of coordination and understanding between the centre and the states. The resources are at a premium and the price for non-compliance is heavy.

There was a healthy balance between centralisation and de-centralisation. Initially, there was greater central play, which helped in stabilising the situation and restoring confidence in the public. Subsequently, the states took on the major role to ensure local adaptation of guidelines. The synergy between the centre and the state contributed significantly in fighting the pandemic.

Though, one hiccup cannot be ignored. The responsibility for procurement of vaccines went from the centre to state to centre. Asking states to go for individual purchases from a common source was sure to land in confusion. This avoidable step was later corrected.

To Conclude

During Covid-19 pandemic, the best of Indian culture and ethos got reflected in the fight against the disease. The strong bonds of the family made sure elderly received adequate care. Local welfare groups came forward to set up oxygen beds and supply food at home to the needy. Public health authorities, initially slow to react, picked up pace quickly. Topping it all were the frontline healthcare professionals who rendered yeoman service to the patients. Medical fraternity as a whole earned the gratitude of the public for going beyond the call of duty. Not to forget the vaccine manufacturers who have risen to the monumental challenge of providing vaccine doses for 1.3 billion countrymen. On the whole, India stands tall among the comity of nations for handling the pandemic crisis.

However, there are many areas, which must be strengthened. Foremost among these is for the country to adopt a national biodefence strategy. This should focus on combatting the current and future bio threats both due to natural causes like a pandemic as well as the due to biological weapon strike.

At the national level, the creation and upgrading of research in life sciences must receive greater attention and resources. Level 4 laboratories need to be created on regional basis. This aspect is closely linked to developing the early warning surveillance systems.

While the public health system exists up to District and Block levels, the equipping and infrastructure deserves immediate attention. The technology has not been embedded into functioning of these setups. The manpower at these places requires training and updating of skills at regular intervals. The communication and decision making process in these nodes requires streamlining.

At the national level, adhoc committees and groups were formed to oversee planning, monitoring and implementation of various decisions. The formal structure for this purpose exists on paper, but did not play an active role. This aspect must be corrected.

Indian defence forces possess, as part of their preparation for biological warfare, considerable know how in managing pandemic like situations. Their potential and expertise should be better harnessed in a similar future crisis.

What Lies Ahead...

There are three main factors that will have a profound influence on the future of biological warfare. These are: type of security threats in the emerging geostrategic environment, advances in molecular sciences and genetic engineering giving rise to the possibility of highly potent and lethal biological agents, and finally, the shadow of Covid-19 pandemic cast in terms of the large number of deaths and the global economic upheaval.

Geostrategic Environment and Nature of Warfare

The geostrategic environment is by itself a product of change with multiple forces at play. The world continues to face same old security threats as well as some new ones. Middle East is in turmoil and the recent developments in Afghanistan hold the potential to destabilise Central Asia. Terrorists, Islamic jihadists, fundamentalists and other non-state actors are active in different parts of the world.

In the new world order, China is posing a serious challenge to the sole super power status of the USA. Equipped with modern war machines, the furious pace of expansion of the Chinese armed forces has raised the heckles of strategists around the globe. China's prowess in conducting research in molecular and genetic sciences is widely recognised. Many of the projects being undertaken in these research facilities meet military requirements. In the coming years, China is expected to be the leader in the field of life sciences and be in a position to develop new generation of biological weapons, if the need be.

China has many security issues like: unification of Taiwan, Uighur unrest in Xinjiang province, subjugation of Tibet, dissatisfaction in Hong Kong, border dispute with India, the control of South China sea and the power rivalry in the Indo-Pacific Ocean. Chinese strategic thought flowing from Sun Tzu focuses on unhinging the enemy by applying coercive force in multiple domains and thus seeking victory that requires no battle. In keeping with the same, China may use a biological weapon surreptitiously to meet a military objective.

It is well established that erstwhile Soviet Union had been running a secret advanced biological weapons program based on gene manipulation and in violation of BTWC 1972. Subsequently, these assets landed with Russia and their current status is uncertain. Clandestine use of biological agents in some of the assassinations carried out by the Russian agents is part of history. Such events to solve inconvenient problems may recur in future.

Even though, the USA has been the target of biological attacks in small measures, it has discontinued the development of biological weapons for offensive use. At the same time, the USA is spearheading the advances in biotechnology through many dedicated research institutes and organisations. This was one of catalytic factor in ensuring fast development of vaccines for SARS CoV-2 virus. Lately, the Centre for Disease Control, USA has proposed a multi-billion dollar research project to develop prototype vaccines for 20 virus families that may spark the next pandemic. A worthwhile effort, but hope it does not turn out to be another "Manhattan" project.

The threat from terrorism continues to grow and will remain critical to global security. Islamic terrorists are active in greater number of countries than ever before. The extremists exploit weak and fragile states. Advances in technology have extended their reach and effect. The recent happenings in Afghanistan have the potential to give further boost to global terrorism.

The terrorist organisations seek to cause large devastation for greater impact and in furtherance of their cause. The attack on the World Trade Centre in New York engineered by Osama bin Laden is one such example. Therefore, WMDs are their first choice and the biological weapons fit the bill becoming the new string in their bow. The incubation delay of the pathogens allows the perpetrators to make good their escape and the viciousness of the disease creates fear and panic among the public. There are suggestions that use of biological weapons by the terrorists in covert operations is imminent. The states will do well to develop preparedness for countering the threat of bioterrorism.

Another related security concern is that of asymmetric warfare undertaken mostly by the weak states and the non-state actors with limited resources. In future, even the major powers like China are likely to prefer other forms of warfare than conventional warfare involving massing of soldiers. Asymmetric warfare strategy hinges on the use of non-conventional weapons and the biological weapons fit the bill eminently. The demonstrative effect of Covid-19 pandemic is likely to inspire many creative thoughts in planning and conduct of asymmetric strategy.

Biological Weapons of the Future

It is well known that the advances in technology drive the changes in warfare. This has happened in a more profound manner in the case of biological warfare. The staggering pace of advances in molecular and genetic sciences have transformed the process of gene modification. It will now be possible to create novel pathogens with specific attributes. Disease causing organisms can now be modified to increase their virulence, transmissibility or resistance to therapeutic interventions.

In addition, the rapid proliferation of biotechnology has ended state monopoly on biological weapons and has increased the access of smaller players to biological weapons development. In future, this will have serious security implications and the world will need to brace up for increase in acts of bioterrorism.

Synthetic biology using tools like CRISPR will be the driver to produce next generation of biological weapons. Apart from targeting the human immune system, the future biological weapons may target the nervous system, genome or microbiome. Also, there is a possibility of recreating the known viruses, which may be extinct now. In future, the face of biological warfare is likely to change with the focus shifting to: binary weapons, agriculture pests, customised agents, biological weapons that do not affect own troops, stealth weapons and weapons with selective targeting capability to target specific race/ethnicity.

Essentially, in future biological weapon development will focus on removing the present shortcomings faced in their employment and at the same time amplify various characteristics. Further, greater push will come from the convergence of technologies like artificial intelligence, robotics and unmanned aerial vehicles for autonomous deployment.

Another point to note is that future biological weapons will mostly be virus based. This is so because the viruses are amenable to gene manipulation and their multiplication rates after entering the host is very high. Even, history supports such an observation as HINI and SARS CoV-2 viruses caused both the pandemics of 1918 and 2019 respectively. So, the proposition is that the virus will be the Brahm Astra of the biological warfare in future.

Next Pandemic

No body knows when the next pandemic may happen, the wisest thing to do is to learn lessons from Covid-19 pandemic and prepare for the eventuality. The world economy will have to develop greater resilience to be able to withstand the shocks of prolonged lock downs. The global logistic supply chains will have to be robust enough to withstand disruptions. The poor states and marginalised sections of the society are the most hit during the pandemic; in future adequate international disaster funding must be made available to them.

Be it a biological war or the pandemic, it will be a joint fight of the military and civilian agencies. In both these situations, contingencies are alike and the best counter-strategy would be to pool the resources and deploy these in an effective and efficient manner. To develop the required degree of jointmanship, top down approach will have to be adopted with a unified command authority.

The world should build on the spectacular success of research scientists in developing vaccines for SARS CoV-2 virus in a record time frame. However, for the good of mankind, international community will have to display greater cooperation in the manufacture and distribution of vaccines. China's reluctance, to facilitate tracing the origin of the coronavirus, has left many gaps in the experts' understanding of the zoonotic transfer of the virus. This casts doubts on the nature and intent of the Chinese biological research programs.

Multilateral Organisations

Covid-19 pandemic exposed many weaknesses and infirmities in the functioning of World Health Organisation (WHO) and International Monetary Fund (IMF). There was lack of diligence on their part to perform the assigned roles and they acted like puppets with the strings being pulled by a major power. Radical changes in their structuring and funding are called for. Major challenges lie ahead for the world with critical exigencies being created by the biological weapons and a future pandemic. Also, there is urgency to disincentivise nations, extremist groups and non-state actors from acquiring and deploying biological weapons. Towards this end, BTWC 1972 must be strengthened for ensuring compliance and enforcement.

Ending with a Note of Caution

There are reasons to believe that at some point in future biological weapons will be used. So, the dictum "prepare or perish" shall apply.

Bibliography

Ainscough MJ, 2002. The Technology of Genetic Engineering Applied to Biowarfare *https://apps.dtic.mil › sti › citations › ADA468243*

Alibek, K., and S. Handelman. 1999. *Biohazard*. New York: Random House.

Alper, J. (1999). From the bioweapons trenches, new tools for battling microbes, Science 284:

American Society for Microbiology (1999). Bioterrorism: frontline response, evaluating U.S. preparedness, March 30, (http://dev. asmusa.org/pasrc/bioterrorismdef.htm)

Anthony H. Cordesman Arleigh A. Burke Chair. Asymmetric and Terrorist Attacks with Biological Weapon, Center for Strategic and International Studies 1800 K Street N.W.Washington, DC 20006

Bill Benson, Colonel U.S. Army. The Evolution of Army Doctrine for Success in the 21st Century

Cole, (1997). The eleventh plague – The politics of biological and chemical warfare ed. Cole, L.A., W.H. Freeman and Company, New York, pgs 289.

Cole, C.A. (1996). The spectre of biological weapons, Scientific American 275:60-65.

Croddy E. Copernicus Books; New York City, NY: 2002. Chemical and Biological Warfare: A Comprehensive Survey for the Concerned Citizen. Google Scholar

Dany Shoham (2015): China's Biological Warfare Programme: An Integrative Study with Special Reference to Biological Weapons Capabilities, Journal of Defence Studies, Vol. 9, No. 2 April-June 2015.

DaSilva, E. Biological warfare, bioterrorism, biodefence and the biological and toxin weapons convention 119.

DaSilva, E.J. and Iaccarino, M. (1999). Emerging diseases: a global threat, Biotechnology Advances 17: 363-384

David P. Clark, Biological Warfare: Infectious Disease and Bioterrorism

Department of Defence (1996). Proliferation: threat and response, April, US Government Printing Office, Washington, D.C.

Department of Foreign Affairs and Trade (1999). Strengthening the biological weapons convention, Australian Biotechnology .

Dobson, R. (1999b). Race hots up to counter bio- terrorism weapons, Innovation —*The Sunday Times*, 15 August.

Domaradskij I.V., Orent L.W. Achievements of the Soviet biological weapons programme and implications for the future. Revue Scientifique et Technique (International Office of Epizootics) 2006;25:153–161. [Google Scholar]]

Drell, S. D., A. D. Sofaer and G. D. Wilson. 1999. *The New Terror: Facing the Threat of Biological and Chemical Weapons*. Stanford, Calif.: Hoover Institution Press.

Ecker, D. and Griffey, R. (1998). Drugs to protect against engineered biological warfare (http://www.ibisrna.com/public/biowar/%2/003.html)

Henderson, D.A. (1999). The looming threat of bioterrorism, Science 283:1279-1281.

J. Kenneth Wickiser, Kevin J. O'Donovan, Michael Washington, Stephen Hummel, F. John Burpo. Engineered Pathogens and Unnatural Biological Weapons: The Future Threat of Synthetic

Biology, *Combating Terrorism Centre Sentinel August 2020*, Volume 13, Issue 8

James Giordano, Department of Neurology, Neuroethics Studies Program, and Program in Brain Science and Global Law and Policy Georgetown University Medical Center, Washington, DC, USA

Jr., E.M. (1997). Biological warfare: a historical perspective http://www.usamriid.army.mil/content/BiowarCourse/H X-3.html)

Kadlec, R. P. (1995). Biological weapons for waging economic warfare. In: Battlefield of the future: 21st century warfare issues, eds. Schneider, B.R. and Grintner, L.E., Department of Defence, Air University, U.S. Department of Defence.

Kaufmann, A.F., Meltzer, M.I. and Schmid, G.P. (1997). The economic impact of a bioterrorist attack: are prevention and post attack intervention programs justifiable? Emerging Infectious Diseases 3:83-94.

Krueger, G.P. and Banderet, L.E. (1997). Effects of chemical protective clothing on military performance: a review of the issues, Military Psychology 9:255-286.

Lederberg, J. 1999. *Biological Weapons: Limiting the Threat.* Cambridge: MIT Press.

Lehrach, H., Bancroft, D. and Maier, E. (1997). Robotics, computing and biology, Interdisciplinary Reviews 22:37- 43.

Lois M. Davis and Jeanne S. Ringel, Public Health Preparedness for Chemical, Biological, Radiological, and Nuclear Weapons

Masato Saito, Natsuko Uchida, Shunsuke Furutani, Mizuho Murahashi, Wilfred Espulgar. *Field-deployable rapid multiple biosensing system for detection of chemical and biological warfare agents* – Microsystems & Nanoengineering (2018)

Michael J. Ainscough, Colonel, USAF. Next Generation Bioweapons: The Technology of Genetic Engineering Applied to Biowarfare And Bioterrorism. *The Counterproliferation Papers Future Warfare Series*

No. 14, USAF Counterproliferation CenterAir War CollegeAir University Maxwell Air Force Base, Alabama, USA

Monath, T.P. and Gordon, L.K. (1998). Strengthening the biological weapons convention, Science 282:1423.

Morse, S. (1998). Defending against biological warfare: programs of defence advanced research projects agency (DARPA). In: Technology and Arms Control for Weapons of Mass Destruction, publ. New York Academy of Sciences, USA,

Nanette J. Pazdernik. Preventing the Use of Biological Weapons: Improving Response Should Prevention Fail

Office of Technology Assessment (1993). Proliferation of weapons of mass destruction: assessing the risks, Washington, D.C., U.S. Government Printing Office.

Pearson, G.S. (1998). The threat of deliberate diseases in the 21st Century (http://www.brad.ac.uk/acad/sbtwc/other/disease.htm)

Preston, R. (1998). Statement before the Senate Judiciary Subcommittee on technology, terrorism and government information, and the select committee on intelligence on chemical and biological weapons threats to America: are we prepared? (http://www.senate.gov/~judiciary/preston.htm)

Preventing the Use of Biological Weapons: Improving Response Should Prevention Fail

Qiao Liang , Wang Xiangsui, 1999. *Un-Restricted Warfare*, People's Liberation Army Literature and Arts Publishing House.

Regis, E. 1999. *The Biology of Doom*. New York: Henry Holt & Co.

Reuben Ananthan Santhana Dass, Bioterrorism: Lessons from the COVID-19 Pandemic, Counter Terrorist Trends and Analsis, Vol 13, Issue 2, March 2021

Rogers, P., Whitby, S. and Dando, M. (1999). Biological warfare against crops, Scientific American 280:70-75.

Ronald M. Atlas, Combating the Threat of Biowarfare and Bioterrorism, BioScience Vol.49 No.6

Russell, P. K. (1999). Vaccines in civilian defence against bioterrorism, Emerging Infectious Diseases 5:498-504.

Schneider, B. R. and Grintner, L. E. (1995). Eds. Battlefield of the Future: 21st Century warfare issues, Air University, U.S. Department of Defence, pgs.287.

Serageldin, I. (1999). Biotechnology and water security in the 21st Century, (http://www.mssrf.orgsg/d99-biotech- water.html)

Steven M. Block, 'The Growing Threat of Biological Weapons', *American Scientist the magazine of Sigma Xi*, The Scientific Research Society

The COVID Crisis: Implications for United States – and Global – Biosecurity.

Thomas V. Inglesby, Tara O'Toole, *From the Center for Civilian Biodefense Studies, Johns Hopkins University School of Medicine*

Thomas V. Inglesby, Tara O'Toole, *From the Center for Civilian Biodefense Studies,* Johns Hopkins *University School of Medicine.*

Tucker, J. B. 2000. *Toxic Terror: Assessing Terrorist Use of Chemical and Biological Weapons.* Cam- bridge: MIT Press.

Index

A

Alpha viruses 16

American Civil War 2

Amerithrax xii, 8

Anthrax 16, 17, 59

Arenaviruses 16

Asymmetric Warfare 55

Aum Shinrikyo xii, 8, 56, 86, 99

B

Bacillis-Calmette-Guerin (BCG) 117

Bacillus Anthracis 17, 59

Bacteria 14, 15

Bascillus Anthracis 3

Battle of Khalkhin Gol 4

Bio Defence Strategy 70

Biological Agents 12, 13, 14, 19, 59

Characteristics 13

Incubation Period 13

Infectivity 13

Lethality 13

Pathogenicity 13

Stability 14

Toxicity 13

Transmissibility 13, 34

Virulence 13, 34

Biological and Toxin Weapons Convention 1972 ix, xiii, 4, 24, 37, 38, 52, 61, 78, 79, 81, 87, 90, 92, 93, 94, 95, 97, 98, 99, 100, 101, 102, 142, 145

Biological Warfare i, iii, vii, ix, 1, 19, 25, 32, 36, 39, 40, 76, 78, 147, 148

Biotechnology xii, xiii, 9, 25, 26, 27, 37, 97, 99, 148, 151

Blue Biotechnology 27

Dark Biotechnology 27

Gold Biotechnology 27

Green Biotechnology 27

Red Biotechnology 26

Yellow Biotechnology 27

Bio Warriors xiii

Black Death 2

Botulinum toxin 7, 8, 16, 18, 56, 85, 90, 92

Botulinum Toxin 59

Braham Astra iii, vii, xiii, 21, 33, 37

C

Centre for Disease Control and Prevention (CDC) 128, 131

Clostridium Botulinum 59

Covid -19 xii, 9, 39, 77, 103, 106, 114, 115, 122

Covishield 123, 124, 125, 133

D

Deoxyribonucleic Acid (DNA) 27

Digital Technologies 51, 75, 136

E

Ebola 16, 32, 51, 56, 59, 87, 91

Encephalitis viruses 17

European wars 2

F

Filoviruses 16

First Sacred War 2

Francisella tularensis 16, 18

Francisella Tularensis 59

Fungi 14, 15

G

Geneva Protocol 4, 79, 84, 85, 93, 94, 98

Genome 29, 32, 34

H

Haemorrhagic fever viruses 80

Hantaviruses 17

I

Influenza Virus 34

Israeli Defence Forces 92

Israel Institute for Biological Research (IIBR) 92

K

Karolstein Castle 3

M

Marburg virus 51, 59, 80

Mutation 28

Mycotoxins 6

N

National Biodefence Strategy 84

National Centre for Disease Control (NCDC) 128, 131

Nipah virus 17

Noborito Institute 5

Nuclear, Biological and Chemical (NBC) xi, 1, 38

Nuclear Warfare 1

O

Ohio River Valley 3

P

Pertussis vaccine 117

Plasmids 29

Pseudomonas pseudomallei 3, 89

R

Retaliatory Assured Destruction (RAD) 42

Ribonucleic Acid (RNA) 29

Rickettsiae 14

S

Salmonella typhimurium 8, 56

SARS-Cov-2 9

SARS CoV-2 xi, xiii, 21, 22, 23, 34, 35, 37, 73, 97, 106, 107, 108, 109, 110, 112, 114, 123, 127, 128, 131, 134, 137, 138, 142, 144

Smallpox 3, 18, 59, 60

Spanish Flu 3, 4, 111, 112

T

Toxins 14, 15, 78

U

Unit 731 4, 81, 83, 85

United Nations Special Commission (UNSCOM) 7, 85

US Army Medical Research Institute of Infectious Diseases (USAMRI-ID) 83, 84

V

Vaccines xiii, 116, 117, 119, 122, 151

Variola major 16, 18

Viruses 14, 15, 30, 32, 33

W

Weapon of Mass Destruction (WMD) 11, 41, 85, 94

World Health Organization 121

X

Xinjiang province 81, 141

www.ingramcontent.com/pod-product-compliance
Lightning Source LLC
LaVergne TN
LVHW051530170726
843492LV00006B/1701